EDUCATING YOUR CLIENTS FROM A TO Z

What to Say and How to Say It

2ND EDITION

NAN BOSS, DVM

© 2011 by Nan Boss

All rights reserved. No part of this publication may be reproduced or transmitted in any form or by any means, electronic or mechanical, including photocopying, recording, or in an information storage and retrieval system, without permission in writing from the publisher. The forms presented in this book were created by Nan Boss, DVM, who is solely responsible for their content. The forms may be reproduced for use by the person purchasing this publication, but may not be sold, transferred, conveyed, or provided to any third party.

The Author and AAHA do not assume responsibility for and make no representation about the suitability or accuracy of the information contained in this Work for any purpose, and make no warranties, either express or implied, including the warranties of merchantability and fitness for a particular purpose. Neither AAHA nor the Author may be held liable for adverse reactions to or damage resulting from the application of this information. Advances in veterinary medicine or practice management may cause information contained herein to become outdated, invalid, or subject to debate by various veterinary or other professionals. AAHA and the Author are not responsible for any inaccuracies, omissions, or editorial errors, nor for any consequence resulting therefrom, including any injury or damage to persons or property. AAHA and the Author shall be held harmless from any and all claims that may arise as a result of any reliance on the information provided. Users should contact their own legal counsel or advisors with respect to the use of this Work or any of the forms in their state prior to implementation.

American Animal Hospital Association Press
12575 West Bayaud Avenue
Lakewood, Colorado 80228
800/252-2242 or 303/986-2800
press@aahanet.org

ISBN-13: 978-1-58326-153-8
Cataloging-in-Publication Data is available from the Library of Congress

Book design by Anita Koury Design
Cover photo: Lifesize/Brand New Images/Getty Images
Printed in the United States of America

11 12 13 / 1 2 3 4 5 6 7 8 9 10

CONTENTS

Introduction v

Veterinary Communication Basics xi

Appointments 1

Behavior and Training 5

Cancer 15

Dentistry 25

Emergencies 37

Fleas and Ticks and Other Things That Bite 43

Grief Counseling and Euthanasia 53

Heartworms 59

Intestinal Parasites 65

Joint Disease 71

Kittens and Puppies 77

Laboratory Testing 89

Money Matters 99

Nutrition and Nutraceuticals 113

Over-the-Counter Sales 123

Pharmacy 129

CONTENTS

Questioning Your Clients 139

Risk Management 149

Surgery and Anesthesia 157

Telephone Skills 171

Urinary Disorders 181

Vaccinations 189

Weight Control and Exercise for Pets 197

X-rays, Ultrasound, and Other High-Tech Procedures 203

Yearly Exams and Senior Health-Care Recommendations 211

Zoonotic Diseases 221

Concluding Thoughts 231

References 233

Index 239

About the Author 247

INTRODUCTION

Hi! I'm Dr. Nan Boss. I own Best Friends Veterinary Center in Grafton, Wisconsin, a town about 20 miles north of Milwaukee.

My practice isn't that big, but about 2,000 clients walk through my doors every year. Along with their pets, my clients bring girlfriends, boyfriends, spouses, children, parents, and friends, which means that I have the opportunity to educate more than 5,000 people about pet care every year: how to choose a pet, what to feed it, how to train it, how to prevent and treat illness, how to care for a pet as it ages, and eventually how to say goodbye.

As a member of the veterinary team, I have an awesome responsibility, as do veterinarians and hospital team members worldwide. How well we communicate the needs of a patient to its owner will in great part determine both the quality and the length of that pet's life. This is true whether we are teaching clients about serious diseases their pets have or teaching them how to avoid a problem in the first place.

Only when there is trust and good communication between pet owners and health-care teams will owners agree to our recommendations. In other words, it doesn't matter how good our clinic's surgeon is if we can't get consent from the owner to have surgery done. The client must first understand why surgery is needed and then trust in the hospital team to do the surgery well. Likewise, our clients won't purchase other services for their pets—such as vaccinations, lab tests, or dental care—if no one explains why they are necessary. If we can't effectively communicate the discharge instructions, the medication dose, or the treatment options, our patients won't be getting the care they deserve.

Whether in sickness or in health, the well-being of our patients is what we are responsible for. Clients don't read medical journals. The only way they will know about new advances in medicine is if we tell them. Sure, they might read something in *Dog Fancy* magazine, and certainly they can find health-care information on the Internet. But we are the most reliable source of health-care information clients have, especially since we can apply what we know to their specific pet. If a pet dies from a disease for which we had a preventive approach or a treatment that we never told the client about, that pet's death is our fault. It is our job to tell clients what products, services, or procedures would benefit their pet. It is their job to decide which ones they want.

According to the American Animal Hospital Association's original 2003 Compliance Study, 35 percent of adult cats are overweight but only 14 percent of clients are told their cats are overweight. According to Antech Laboratories, 87 percent of veterinarians do senior wellness testing on their own pets, yet only 9 percent offer it to their clients. The Compliance Study also revealed that 70 percent of pet owners had never heard of senior screening. According to Hill's, a pet nutrition company, only 7 percent of pets who could benefit from a therapeutic diet are eating one. The reason these numbers are so low is that we are not spending the time and effort that we should in teaching our clients about proper care for their pets.

The only way we can excel as health-care professionals, no matter how much we care about our patients, is to be skilled in relating to their owners. Therefore, the roles of veterinary employees are evolving, with client education and liaison becoming a top priority for all team members, both at the front desk and in the exam rooms. Doctors shouldn't need to perform 5,000 repetitions of "the dental talk" or "the flea talk." Trained and knowledgeable employees can and should help educate clients and promote veterinary services. Client relations specialists (CRSes), technicians, and assistants are critical to a clinic's success.

Unfortunately, most team members, including the veterinarians, have little or no training in communication, teaching, or public relations. Communicating well with clients requires skills that need to be developed, nurtured, and practiced. Some people are naturally gifted in this area while others may have to work harder at it. Anyone, whether bold or shy, bubbly or reserved, outspoken or tongue-tied, can learn to communicate more effectively with clients.

Moreover, doctors aren't taught how to do client education in veterinary school. Although 35 to 50 percent of our patients are overweight or obese (depending on what study you use), for example, the average veterinarian receives just 1.5 hours of class time on obesity management while in veterinary school. Obesity not only leads to cancer, orthopedic problems, diabetes, and hepatic lipidosis but also reduces a pet's life expectancy by an estimated two to three years. Yet little emphasis in school usually translates to little emphasis in the exam room, so far too few clients truly understand the health risks or the best remedies for obesity. For most of the other topics in this book it's the same story: Insufficient training leads to insufficient teaching, which in turn leads to a lower quality of patient care.

Many veterinary hospitals schedule 15- to 20-minute exams—not enough time for client education. Taking more time for exams and wellness visits almost always improves the average transaction fee (ATF) as well as the healthcare information provided to the client. Longer appointment times may be necessary to improve the client education delivered in your hospital, but this need not mean more demands on the doctors' time. Other team members can provide support by communicating important guidelines and recommendations, explaining the reasoning behind them, and answering clients' questions.

Every client visit, in fact, provides multiple opportunities for team members to communicate and reinforce important information. But the time we have with clients is often not well spent. Sometimes it's because we don't have a protocol or a system that ensures that every client receives consistent information. Many times we assume clients know things that they actually don't have a clue about (like the pet is too fat!), so we miss opportunities to remedy the situation. Sometimes it's because we are just plain poor communicators. We may sound critical or a little negative instead of being positive, upbeat, and friendly.

The nice thing about communication skills is that much of it can be learned, and what we learn is timeless. No matter what new drug or technology comes along, the ways to interact with clients and coworkers successfully do not change. Skillful communication with people is the key to excellence in the workplace now and will remain so in the future.

The time and effort we invest in learning communication techniques will be well spent. According to Zig Ziglar, a motivational speaker and author of several books on interpersonal skills, just 15 percent of success at any job results from technical skills. The remaining 85 percent results from people skills. No matter how smart we were in school, our education alone will only get us 15 percent of the way to being a valuable addition to a practice team. In fact, in our employers' eyes, our attitude, effort, willingness to change and grow on the job, and ability to communicate well with all types of people are our most important assets. Our clients don't know what our grade point average was or how many hours we've devoted to continuing education, but they sure notice if we aren't gentle with their pets, don't pay attention to them when they speak, or can't explain to them why their pet needs a new vaccine.

This book will enable you to acquire that other 85 percent of effectiveness that Ziglar was talking about. Whether you are a veterinary student, a veterinary technician, a veterinary assistant, or part of the front-office team, you will find great information here that you can put to use on a day-to-day basis. Remember that the entire team will be more successful if everyone is speaking to the client with one voice. If all team members read and discuss the concepts in this book, it can jump-start a collaborative effort. As you read, determine what your role is in client education and think about which concepts you may want to discuss with others on your team.

The opening sections of the book introduce valuable communication strategies that you can put into practice immediately. Learning new communication skills will likely be an ongoing process, and you will want to return to this section again and again to review and practice the skills described. In the "A to Z" sections of the book, you will find tips on communicating with clients on a broad range of issues. This book covers everything from appointments to zoonotic diseases. Whether you are dealing with a pet emergency, explaining high-tech procedures like X-rays and ultrasounds, or simply want to know how to communicate more effectively with clients on the telephone, you will find it in these sections. This book also contains many helpful client handouts and forms, which you can feel free to modify and use in your own practice. For your convenience, they are provided on this book's accompanying website, www.aahanet.org/EYC.

I hope this book prods you to grow and excel and that it helps everyone at your practice to work together as a team. Interpersonal relationships, between team members as well as between clients and the team, can become top-notch with these techniques, and ultimately, the quality of pet care will be top-notch as well.

VETERINARY COMMUNICATION BASICS

Communicating with clients may be one of the most enjoyable parts of your job and one of the most intimidating. Even if you consider yourself a "people person" as much as a "dog person" or a "cat person," it's undeniable that working with people can be a challenge. In this section, I will provide you with tips that will enable you to convey a contagious positive attitude to the clients who enter the practice, that will help you increase their understanding of how to care for their pets, and that will allow you to show empathy and lend your support to clients when needed.

You will be educating clients about a host of issues—such as the ones discussed in the "A to Z" section of this book—so before we look at those specific topics, let's examine the rules of good communication skills. Below I discuss 16 maxims for good communication, and then we will look at the two main types of education you will likely be doing and the steps involved in each opportunity to educate. You may find it helpful to come back to this section again later so that you can refresh your memory. Practice the skills described until they are second nature to you, and you will find that you are more of a "people person" than you knew.

THE EXCELLENT COMMUNICATOR: 16 MAXIMS

Communicating well with veterinary clients starts with some basic rules. I will first discuss these maxims and later show how they apply in real-life situations. Because these ideas are so important to good client education, you'll see them repeated throughout this book. When the maxims appear on the pages of later chapters, let them serve as reminders to you to enlist the skills you have learned here.

1. The Entire Team Must Be Great Communicators!

One person alone cannot handle all client educational needs in a veterinary practice. Good client communication is a team effort, and every team member—from the front-office team to the doctors to the kennel attendants—must be conveying the same messages. Everyone on the team must be able to express that your hospital is a place where owners and patients are enjoyed and respected. Just one team member who conveys an uncaring attitude or gives misinformation can spoil a client's experience.

Good communication with other team members is also essential. Respect and courtesy for each other are basic requirements for anyone on the clinic team. Before they can be effective with clients, all team members must first be able to talk to each other about what messages need to be sent to the clients.

A team, by definition, is two or more people working together to reach common goals. What are your clinic's goals? Until you know, you can't work with other team members to meet them, nor can you give clients the service they want and deserve. All members of the team who have client communication as part of their job description (which is everyone on the team!) must be on the same page about a host of issues, or clients will end up being confused because they were told different things by different people. Should all cats be vaccinated for feline leukemia, or just those that go outdoors, or those in multi-cat households? What pet foods do you recommend and why? When should you recommend pre-anesthetic blood testing or a stool check? Before you discuss or promote specific protocols with your clients, you need to know what those protocols are. If the practice does not yet have a systematic set of protocols for all team members to express to clients, the team leaders may wish to consult *How We Do Things Here*, published by AAHA Press. It shows veterinary practice owners and managers how to develop their hospital's medical and service protocols, from client education to vaccinations, and then train the whole team so clients get a consistent message.

What else does your clinic want to communicate to clients, and how? Do you want to emphasize high-tech medicine, or attentive service? Do you want to see more clients quickly, or fewer clients with longer appointments? Do you want to expand services for birds or exotic species, specialize in dental services, or stick to the basics of general practice? All such goals should be communicated to the team at all levels so that everyone can be headed in the same direction.

On a day-to-day level there are additional considerations. How should you answer the phone? What are the clinic's policies on billing or making payments? How much freedom do you have to give refunds or exchanges? When is it all right to handle a problem yourself, and when should you call a supervisor to help you? Veterinary clinics need to have service protocols and communication protocols so that each member of the team knows his or her role for a particular service, like vaccinations, as well as what is appropriate and necessary to say to clients at these times.

Consistency is important for any office to run smoothly. Clients feel secure when team members are uniform in their approach and advice. In turn, as a team member you will feel secure when you know exactly what to say or recommend to clients. Creating protocols and guidelines for patient care and technical procedures is an essential part of this process. Proper training and follow-up also are needed to ensure that each employee knows what is expected and imparts the right information to the clients.

Obviously, there is more to successful communication than meets the eye. Hopefully, your clinic has an office manual and regular team meetings, and all team members are familiar with the goals and aspirations of the practice's managers or owners. If not, doctors and managers should be consulted and should work together to make progress in this area. Developing a set of protocols and making sure everyone makes use of them is an ongoing process in which everyone participates. All team members can provide input, help develop these policies, and update them as needed so that the whole team can be more effective. Care recommendations and payment policies should be in writing so that any team member, new or experienced, can give the same information to every client.

If you and your team members take the time to improve communication with clients and to develop, use, and promote a client-education program, you can practice better medicine. You will be taking better care of your clients and their pets, and you will also earn more money for your hospital. Good veterinary team members must learn to be good communicators, educators, and salespeople if they are to provide good pet care, because you can't help the pet if you can't get through to the owner.

2. Remember the Golden Rule: Treat Your Clients as You Would Wish to Be Treated—or Better, Exceed Their Expectations!

There's no substitute for old-fashioned hospitality. I've found that one of the best ways to start off on a good footing with clients—whether it's the first time they've visited the office or the tenth—is for the front-office team to treat them as if they were guests in their home. Offer to hang up their coats, serve them coffee, help them out to the car, or do anything else that can be done to make them feel welcome and appreciated. The entire team can follow suit as the clients go through the different stages of the visit.

You clean your house when you are expecting company, and your hospital should be clean as well. You encourage guests to return again, and you should ask your clients to as well: "Please come visit us again!" can be said with a genuine attitude that shows that you mean it.

Keep this in mind as well:

If we take people as we find them, we may make them worse
but, if we treat them as though they are what they should be,
we help them to become what they are capable of becoming.

—JOHANN WOLFGANG VON GOETHE

This means that most people will rise to the level of our expectations. Don't patronize people or judge them by their appearance. Talk to your clients as intelligent adults who will make intelligent decisions. Pet owners have the right and responsibility to make decisions for their pets' care. Your job is to give them the information and help they need to make good choices. Expect the best from your clients, and most of them will meet your expectations.

Unfortunately, there will be a few clients who will not be receptive to what you are trying to teach. As any educator can tell you, not all students come to class equally prepared to learn. You will have "A student" clients and those who are disruptive or disinterested. You will have tardy clients, ones who cut class, and those who don't do their homework, don't pay attention to the teacher, or need help understanding. Be prepared to go the extra mile for any client who is willing to listen and learn. Don't sweat the clients who aren't engaged. Invest your time and effort where it's most likely to pay off—on the clients who care about their pets and want to take good care of them.

This doesn't mean you should be rude to those who don't want first-class service. It just means you need to maintain perspective, focus on the positive, and don't let yourself get dragged down by a few underachieving pet owners. "A negative attitude cancels all positive skills" is my mantra for remembering this principle.

3. Look and Act Professional

When you are talking to a client, you are giving a performance. You are not acting—you are not pretending to be someone else—but you are performing for an audience. The effectiveness of your presentation will depend on how your audience perceives you. Your dress, speech, and mannerisms will all be key factors in making you seem credible—or not.

In other words, like it or not, people will judge you on your appearance. If you want to be accorded the respect deserving of a professional person and be listened to as an expert, you must look the part. Wear clean scrubs or a lab coat with a name badge. Introduce yourself politely. Don't swear. Speak proper English.

Clients will notice your body language and posture. They will also notice if you make eye contact, listen actively (nodding or saying "I see" or "mm-hmm" in response to what he or she is saying), and articulate well. Be sure you enter an exam room prepared: Have the correct file and any appropriate handouts with you, know the name and sex of the pet, and have an extra pen for the owner to use if any forms need to be filled out or signed.

Be prompt. Chronically running behind schedule communicates inefficiency and poor service. If team members often keep clients waiting, it's time to revamp your appointment system. The number one complaint of patients about physicians who treat humans, according to the book *Listen to Me, Doctor: Taking Charge of Your Own Health Care,* by Marti Ann Schwartz, is "long waits for appointments," and clients probably feel the same about their veterinarians. Waiting time is also a primary reason clients switch from one practice to another.

You must also remember your manners. The number three complaint in Schwartz's book is "doctors who don't introduce themselves." Number four is "doctors who don't apologize for being late." Minding your manners is important for all team members, not just the doctors.

Take a good, hard look at yourself, your clinic, and other team members and how you are presenting your clinic and your profession. Even though the points just listed sound like the common courtesies everyone knows, it's surprising how many times they are not observed. How does your practice appear to a customer? If your scrub top or lab coat is dirty, will your clients think your surgery room is clean? If you still dress like a high school or college student, will your clients respect you, or will they treat you like a student? And if you haven't updated your hairstyle in 15 years (or your waiting room, for that matter), why would your clients think your knowledge is up-to-date?

This doesn't mean you can't be yourself or you shouldn't have a sense of humor. Be professional, but keep in mind that clients don't get pets to ponder the great truths of the universe. They get them because they are cute and fun. It doesn't demean the profession to wear a scrub top or lab coat with little kitties on it or to enjoy the puppies and kittens that come through the door.

The art of performing for clients is to speak to them conversationally, as if they were your friends, while behaving with the utmost professionalism and using phrases you've practiced and used many times before. To make clients feel "talked to," not "talked at," you have to engage them in discussion, listen to their replies, and steer the conversation where you want it to go. Sounds like a lot to ask, doesn't it? With practice, however, you can do it, and you will find it to be very rewarding.

4. Rehearse!

You won't give a flawless performance without rehearsals. A successful performer—whether an actor, a business or marketing professional, or a salesperson—comes to a business meeting or sales call rehearsed and prepared.

If you were the vice president of Boeing and were flying off to Europe for a sales presentation to a European airline that might purchase millions of dollars' worth of planes, you'd work pretty hard at that presentation, wouldn't you? You'd rehearse and prepare, have all your charts and graphs and figures ready, and make sure you were well rested and dressed appropriately.

Obviously, you are not a Boeing vice president; however, you are making dozens of small presentations to clients every day. Your performances are going to determine the amount of money in the clinic's till at the end of the day and the amount of pride and satisfaction you derive from your day's work. Have you rehearsed your lines? Are you using the most effective words and phrases? Are you practicing how to respond to irate, confused, or stubborn clients?

It helps to role-play with other team members and make cue cards with scripts for selling wellness packages, surgery price quotes, or other clinic services. You will feel much more confident and in control when you know exactly what to say.

It is not demeaning or silly to think of your job as a series of sales pitches or performances you put on for your clients. Practicing or rehearsing lines doesn't make you insincere, as long as you still believe in what you are selling. Being prepared provides security. It is much easier to take on a role and say your lines than to talk to clients unrehearsed. In fact, it will provide you much pleasure to know that if you give a good presentation, your patients will get the care they deserve.

It's important to remember that clients can easily tell the difference between a "canned speech" and an informative conversation. Make sure your rehearsal doesn't interfere with the quality of your message. Have an underlying belief in the value of the care you are offering to the client, as well as a sincere interest in both the client and the patient. Always remember what you are really talking about—the health and happiness of a treasured pet.

5. Communicate That You Are Happy and Enjoying Your Work

No one wants to interact with crabby, rude, or depressed people. Clients also don't have the slightest interest in your problems. So no matter how lousy or stressed you feel, put on a smile when you come to work!

Did you know that if you enjoy what you do, you will live longer? (George 2006). Happiness at work is the most accurate predictor of life expectancy. It is more accurate even than such risk factors as smoking and obesity. It's also true that the physical act of smiling actually releases neurotransmitters that elevate your mood. The more you smile, the happier you will become.

If you pass me on the road when I'm driving to work each morning, you'll see me driving along with a big smile on my face. I'm trying to release those happy neurotransmitters before I get to the clinic. Did you ever notice how you can be in a really bad mood, but if you make a big effort to talk and interact cheerfully with clients for five or ten minutes, by the time they leave you're in a good mood again? That's those neurotransmitters at work.

People are more likely to be happy in a cheerful environment. Some colors have been shown to make you feel more upbeat while others can literally make you feel "blue." Keep your decor, pictures, and scrubs or lab coats bright, clean, and cheery. Joke with your coworkers and your clients. Keep flowers on the counter, cartoons on the bulletin board, and snacks in the lunchroom. Put pictures of your pets and your clients' pets on the wall. Try replacing your regular fluorescent lightbulbs with full-spectrum bulbs—they have been shown to help prevent depression and seasonal affective disorder.

Show your clients you like their animals as well. Pet the cat. Let the dog lick your face. One of the main ways to keep clients coming back is to make it obvious that you like what you are doing. Clients are also more likely to follow your recommendations when it's clear you care about your patients on a personal level.

Don't let yourself become burned-out on the job. If you truly don't like what you are doing, you owe it to yourself to find a career you like better—before you make yourself and others around you miserable. If you are happy with what you do but are simply stale or have that "been there, done that" feeling, the cure is simple. Learn something new or do something different! There is always something exciting happening in veterinary medicine. Go to a seminar, read a few good books, or learn a new skill. If your clinic provides continuing education assistance, you should take advantage of it. You owe it to yourself and your clients to stay interested, involved, and up-to-date.

Communicate to your clients that you enjoy them, their pets, and your work and they will reward you with affection and loyalty. Communicate that you don't care, are having a bad day, or don't like their pets, and clients are likely to go elsewhere.

6. Don't Get Defensive

Good customer service representatives don't have to be right. It is never productive to get into arguments with clients. Customers may not always be right but they are always the customer. Make them feel good, important, or clever and they will come back to your clinic. Make them feel wrong, stupid, or small and you will lose them.

It is always better, and much less costly, to retain a client than to recruit a new one. Not only will angry clients go elsewhere, but they will also tell a dozen other people about the poor service they received, losing you additional clients as well. After a client has left, you have lost the opportunity to help his or her pet get the good care your clinic provides. You have also lost the opportunity to turn that client into a better client, meaning a more educated pet owner.

Assume that your clients come to your office with good intentions, that they care about their pets, and that they will try to take good care of them. Don't assume that their goal for the day is to make your life miserable! Don't try to prove your superiority or your knowledge. Don't force your client to give in. Being humble and letting the client win is usually the best strategy.

It is easy to interpret clients' questions as threatening when they are not. For example, "I don't understand the bill" may sound like "You overcharged me," but it isn't. The client who says, "Boy, this dog sure costs me a lot of money" may be bragging to other people in the waiting room about how much he or she can afford to spend, rather than criticizing the bill. Do not read things into clients' comments that are not really there.

If a client says, "You people don't know what you are doing," it is much more constructive to say, "I can see how it might look that way. Let me see what I can do to solve the problem" than it is to say, "If you don't like it, get lost." Don't take things personally if you can help it, and don't make excuses.

7. Listen to the Client

Listening is the other half of good communication. "Doctors who don't listen" is also on the list of complaints in Schwartz's book. You need to understand the client's concerns and make sure you are answering all his or her questions. Read his or her body language and practice active listening skills. Don't fall into the habit of thinking about your next question; pay attention to the answer the client is giving. Even though you think you've heard it all before, and you may have, for that client it's a new story and you need to pay attention.

Allow the client to be comfortable enough to ask the "stupid" (but important) questions. If you seem hurried or impatient, the client may not ask you what he or she needs to know. The pet won't receive the care it should if the owner does the wrong thing or doesn't obtain important information that affects its treatment.

If a pet owner refuses care, you need to ask the owner why and then listen carefully so you can deal with his or her concerns. The client may have a fear of anesthesia for the pet, may not realize that you are willing to work out a payment plan, or may misunderstand the expected outcome of a procedure.

Ask lots of questions. Most clients are very happy—and even flattered—to answer your questions about their pets' lifestyles so you can recommend needed care. They want you to be clear and explain what is available. Once you've asked a question, wait for the client to think and reply.

Asking questions and simply waiting for the client to answer seems simple enough, but I've found it may be difficult to do this at first. At first it may seem awkward and rude to just stand there and look at the client after you've asked a question. But resist the temptation to always fill in the silence with conversation. The client may need a moment as he or she ponders the question, and if you are waiting it communicates that you are truly interested in what he or she has to say.

It takes time, effort, training, and—again—rehearsals to learn to be an advocate for your patients, to come right out and ask the client what you need to know. You and the rest of the team need to practice saying things like "Is there a particular reason you don't wish to schedule this dental now?" You can't address the client's concern about anesthesia, or fees, or whatever is bothering him or her, if you don't know what the problem is. And you can't give the client the services and products he or she needs if you don't know what they are.

8. Be Honest with Your Clients and Don't Surprise Them

Here are two more complaints from *Listen to Me, Doctor*: "doctors who 'sugar coat' the truth about treatment, procedures, or diagnoses" and "high fees or unexplained fees."

Never beat around the bush with your clients. If an animal is in pain or a procedure will be painful, tell the client. Then explain how you can help. If an animal is dying, explain how and when that might happen so the client can deal with it. If a procedure will be expensive, discuss it up-front so the client can budget or plan accordingly. Explain what you want to do, why you want to do it, and how much it will cost. (See the "Money Matters" section of this book for more information on providing detailed estimates for your clients.)

Clients want and deserve to know the whole truth—every client, every time.

9. Be Enthusiastic and Creative

Show your clients how interesting and exciting medicine and physiology can be. Show your enthusiasm for the latest and greatest treatments.

I find nature endlessly fascinating. Did you know that fleas can hop so well because they have a little superball above their hind legs, made of the most elastic substance known? What a cool thing! Isn't it amazing that skin can stretch to accommodate swelling or pregnancy and then return to its original shape? Isn't it awesome that sparrows can go through an entire winter without their little feet freezing and falling off?

Animals are amazing. So are benchtop and handheld chemistry machines, ultrasound scanners, and modern anesthetics. Another item on the list of complaints about physicians is "doctors who refuse to talk about new medicines or treatments." Make sure your clients appreciate how complicated the body is and how amazingly sophisticated modern veterinary medicine can be. Your clients want to know you're up-to-date.

I often use trivia to illustrate my points when discussing pet care. *Ripley's Believe It or Not* was the most popular book in my waiting room for years, until it finally fell apart. Try to use trivia, fun facts, and quizzes to make your educational efforts hit home.

It also helps to tie animal health to human health. For instance, when discussing dental care with clients, I tell them what I read in *Cosmopolitan* magazine—that pregnant women with periodontal disease are seven times more likely to have a premature or low-birth-weight baby (Torpy et al. 2008). Maybe if it does that to people, it's not good for dogs either. Dental disease is a serious matter, not just a cosmetic problem.

Clients like knowing how high fleas can hop, how fast greyhounds can run, and how big heartworms are. Keep in mind that people have pets because they're fun. Try to make learning about their care fun as well. Shows like those on Animal Planet are filled with such facts, and that is what makes them so popular. Use trivia and fun facts, and tie animal health to human health, and you'll have your clients tuning in to hear what you have to say.

10. Remember, Different People Learn Best in Different Ways

Some of your clients are visual learners, some are auditory, and some need to touch or feel to learn. If you aren't getting through to a client by talking, try a handout, a DVD, or a dental or skeletal model. Learn to be flexible in your teaching methods so you can reach more of your clients. Be creative. If your presentation or speech doesn't seem to be as effective as you'd like, change it and try a different approach.

Visual people tend to speak very quickly. They use visual phrases like "I see" or "See you later." They learn best by reading and writing, so they often take notes or make lists in order to remember things. Although written materials are useful for any style, they are particularly helpful for visual communicators (Semb and Ellis 1994; Sisson et al. 1992).

Auditory communicators speak at a moderate rate. They are more likely to use phrases such as "I hear you" or "Talk to you later." They learn well from lectures or audiotapes and are less likely to take notes. Although they will usually get more out of an exam room discussion than other styles of presenting the topic, they also are easily distracted by the barking dog or crying cat in the next room.

Kinesthetic communicators are "slow talkers." They think before they speak, and they use a lot of gestures. They will miss a lot of what a visual, fast-talking person says—it may seem like babbling to them. When I need to speak with kinesthetic people, I take a deep breath and slow myself down when I enter the exam room. If I talk too quickly, I may lose them. When training kinesthetic people, you need to be hands-on. They can't learn how to give their cat a pill from your description; they have to actually try it. Their verbal responses may be phrases such as "Catch you later" or "I get it."

Often you don't know what type of personality or communication style your client has, so here's another way to accommodate for different styles. About half the population likes to receive information in the form of stories. The other half prefers facts and figures. If you aren't sure, combine a fact with a feeling or a story with a statistic. For example, when talking about dental care, you could say, "Dogs live two to three years longer when they receive good dental care. After we clean her teeth, Molly will feel so much better." That's a fact (longer life expectancy) combined with a feeling (emphasizing how Molly will feel and the bond between the owner and the pet).

No matter what style of learning a pet owner needs, if you think ahead and plan what you are going to say to incorporate different types of information, you are more likely to have your message hit home. Use pictures whenever possible. Even nonvisual people remember pictures better than words. Try not to speak too quickly or too slowly. A medium speed is best when you don't know whether the client is visual, auditory, or kinesthetic.

Whatever handout or material you use, explain why you want your clients (or team members) to read or watch it. If you stress its importance, they are more likely to pay attention than if you simply hand it to them without comment. Use a phrase such as "The doctor thinks it's very important that you read (or watch) this," or "This sheet explains why our hospital recommends this procedure." Remember that the client has come to your hospital for your expert opinion and knowledge of pet health care. If you think a client may be auditory or kinesthetic, go ahead and give him or her the handout, but don't stop there. Maybe that client would do better with a video or a model. Take the time to offer this alternative, so that you are communicating the information in a way that will be effective.

11. Repetition Is Key!

The average person needs to hear about a product or service at least five times before he or she will purchase it. This is called the Repetition Rule of Marketing. Five times! (Multiply your number of clients by five, plus add a few more for spouses and other family members—no wonder you're tired of saying the same thing!) Start talking about long-term care needs early, so by the time the pet needs that care, the owner is comfortable with the idea.

Let's use dental care as an example again. Say you have 1,000 clients. Each needs to hear about dental care five times. That's 5,000 repetitions. And that's just one disease.

Mention dental care to new puppy or kitten owners at their very first visit. At their second visit, give them a sample of toothpaste and a tooth-brushing

---

GETTING YOUR MESSAGE ACROSS

According to research by Edgar Dale and the National Training Laboratory Institute for Applied Behavioral Science, after hearing a lecture, people remember only 5 percent of the information, on average. When reading, they retain about 10 percent. When the material is audiovisual, such as in a video, the retention rate is 20 percent. When a demonstration is given, it is 30 percent, and with discussion-group learning, it is 50 percent. Practice by doing is much better, 75 percent, and when someone has to teach others or apply information immediately in a real situation, the retention rate is 90 percent. That is why it makes so much sense to do more than just tell your clients how to perform a new skill: Demonstrate the skill, and then have them perform it, for example. They will not only retain the information better, they will also feel more confident.

It is also crucial to send written materials home about anything that's important and to mention pet-care needs and services multiple times. No matter how good your presentation is, your client is not going to remember it the first time. When possible, show videos, demonstrate, have the client demonstrate for you, or ask him or her to repeat back what you said.

Also, keep in mind that the person in the room is often not the only, or even the primary, caregiver for the pet. You may talk about dental care to Ms. Jones this year, and have to start all over again with Mr. Jones next year. (Here's a helpful tip: Always record who brings the pet in for each visit so you know who's heard what during previous visits.) Try to educate all the family members, or the pet may not get the care you hope for when it gets home.

demonstration. At every annual visit, mention the future need for dental care. By the time the pet is four or five years old and ready for its first prophylactic treatment, the client will be ready as well.

Use the same technique with senior screening tests, pre-anesthetic panels, heartworm prevention, and flea control. Don't wait until the last minute to educate your clients about their pets' needs.

Another way to think of this is to realize that even motivated people remember less than 20 percent of what they hear. That's why everyone took notes on school lectures—even though the material was important, by the next week no one could remember most of it unless one wrote it down and studied it. In the exam room with a tense pet owner, a nervous pet, and perhaps several screaming children, you will be lucky to achieve 20 percent retention. Do not expect your clients to remember anything you have told them. If they do, assume it will be the wrong thing, such as the fact that Buffy yelped when you poked her with that needle, or exactly how many minutes they had to wait for you to come to the room.

12. Use Simple Language

Unless you know the client is a physician, nurse, or other medical professional, assume he or she doesn't know medical terminology. Did you know that 42 percent of people in the United States never read a book again after they graduate from high school or college? (Hawk and Shah 2007). Most people don't know Earth goes around the sun once a year, much less how a vaccine works. Many will never read anything you give them and will surrender a dog to a humane society long before they ever go to the library and take out a book on obedience training. On the other hand, veterinary medicine is growing more and more sophisticated, and some of your clients are, too. Your "A" clients probably know a great deal about pet health care. How do you manage to treat both types of clients appropriately?

Take this as a challenge. You need to simplify without sounding patronizing. If you see a blank look on the client's face, take a step back and try again. If the client looks bored, jump ahead a little. Many veterinarians and technicians, especially new graduates, spend more time trying to impress the clients than they do educating them. A common complaint about physicians treating people, again from Schwartz's book, is "doctors who use medical jargon and don't provide written information," which brings me to the next point.

13. Write It Down!

Send your clients home with quality, professional, easy-to-read materials. They will appreciate your efforts on their behalf. Remember that your best clients are your most educated clients and vice versa.

Client education is especially important with serious diseases like Cushing's disease or hyperthyroidism. Clients should learn about and understand their pets' diseases, just as you would expect them to educate themselves about their own health. A disease diagnosis forces clients to make decisions about their pets' care, so they need something solid to go on.

Good handouts can be purchased from many sources. With the availability of commercial handouts and DVDs, easy-to-use word-processing software, high-quality copiers and scanners, and copy stores that can scan in and modify any document or picture, there is no longer any need to send home low-quality handouts. Unfortunately, many of the client-education handouts and pamphlets available through computer software systems, or from drug suppliers, are too simple or too promotional of a particular brand or product. It is usually better to spend a few dollars to purchase good handouts or make your own. Many free forms and client handouts are available at the website of *DVM360 Newsmagazine* (www.dvm360.com). The American Animal Hospital Association has brochures for sale on the topics of pet health, pet behavior, and pet loss as well as a host of other helpful materials and client forms.

Don't assume your clients won't read the materials you give them. More and more, clients are taking an active role in researching their pets' health issues just as they are with their own health issues. Some clients will go so far as to download and read 120 pages of research material on feline infectious peritonitis (FIP) from the Internet. In fact, up to one-third of veterinary clients in a Wisconsin Veterinary Medical Association survey said they got their primary veterinary health-care information from the Internet. Some of this information is valuable; some of it is quackery. Many clients can't tell the difference. Volunteer as much educational material as your clients seem to want, because you don't know what kind of information—or misinformation—they will find on their own. Refer them specifically to good websites with reliable information and provide links to those sites on your own website.

Luckily, only a few clients can't read or don't understand anything you give them or tell them. Most clients are somewhere in between. They will read at least some of the materials you give them, and they will gain an appreciation for their pets' treatment needs if you take the time to explain things and coach them. These clients will then go on to be more conscientious pet owners because they understand their pets' needs.

ADVANTAGES OF WRITTEN MATERIALS

Why provide written handouts to your clients? There are many reasons. Here is a summary of some of the benefits:

1. People remember a very small portion of what they hear. When they have written handouts, they can review the information at home.
2. The person in the exam room with you isn't always the only one who helps care for the pet. Others in the family who care for the pet can read the information that you send home.
3. Having written material available makes all team members look more knowledgeable and professional.
4. Using handouts and forms consistently ensures you are giving the same information to every client, no matter which doctor or other team member sees the client, and no matter how tired or distracted you are.
5. Clients become more aware of the knowledge and services you can offer their pets when the written materials are well done.
6. Clients will comply better with your recommendations if they understand why you are making those recommendations. In other words, if they don't understand what medication is going to do for their pets, they may not administer the pills. When you reinforce your recommendations with written materials, the compliance rate is higher.
7. Anything you send home or mail to the client strengthens the bond between you and the client and promotes the practice.

Never let clients leave without a handout. You can adapt materials from articles you read, use brochures from drug companies, or purchase or copy handouts from other sources. (See Resources at the end of this section.) Try to add your clinic name to every handout and see if you can tailor the information to your area, practice methods, and style. Handout sources for the "A to Z" topics in this book are listed with each topic.

At my clinic, all handouts on common specific diseases are kept in tabbed folders in file cabinet drawers located in the checkout area. The folder has the name of the handout on the tab and a maximum and minimum amount of that handout to print on the front. When a folder is nearly empty, I take it out and put it in a tray for someone to restock. They know how many to make or order by the numbers on the front of the folder. Handouts we don't use as often are printed out only as needed.

Anytime my patients come in for a routine visit, such as for annual exams and vaccinations or heartworm testing, we ask their owners to read a handout while waiting for the doctor or technician. Even when they just set it on the seat next to them and don't read it, the handout opens the door for us to discuss that topic. Client-education DVDs and websites also work well for this purpose, and many good ones are available. Both handouts and videos help occupy clients' time while waiting, and they spark discussions about new topics. Make learning about animal care fun!

Your clients won't buy products and services from you—and therefore won't take the best possible care of their pets—if they don't know what's available. The more information clients get from you, the healthier your patients will be, and the longer they will live.

Good handouts and forms and written hospital protocols not only help you communicate better with your clients, but also improve team education and communication and provide more efficient patient care when pets are in the hospital.

This brings me to lawsuits and liability. Good communication can sometimes save a clinic from disaster. Give clear written instructions and make sure your client knows what disease his or her pet has and how it is diagnosed and treated. Attaching handouts to line items in your computer system, such as vaccine releases and medication information sheets, ensures that these will be printed and given to clients consistently. Any procedure or product that has risks associated with it deserves use of written materials. Be sure you are providing good, accurate estimates and updates on charges for hospitalized pets, so there are no misunderstandings later. Make sure clients also know their payment options before treatment begins.

Sometimes clients come in for a second opinion who have no idea what disease their pets have or what the prescribed medication is supposed to actually do. In those cases, we can request the pet's records from the original veterinarian. However, you do not want your own clients to leave your office uninformed. Your hospital team is responsible for educating clients about their pets' care and treatments. If a pet dies of a disease that could have been prevented with a vaccine that your client was never informed about, your team hasn't done its job. On the other hand, if you gave the client a handout on the disease and he or she chose not to purchase that vaccine, you are no longer responsible if the pet gets sick.

It can take a long time to develop an effective style of communication and to learn to establish a rapport with your clients. Good handouts and written materials help to compensate for any deficiencies in your verbal communication. They help you to teach your clients what they should know about pet care, and they enrich and strengthen the bond between you and the client.

14. Think of Yourself as a Teacher

Did it ever occur to you when you were in school that to be a veterinary medical professional was to be a teacher? The only way you can take good care of your patients is to educate their owners on how to take care of them. In fact, the better you are at teaching, the better you are at practicing medicine or assisting the veterinarian for whom you work.

Your clients don't know what your grade point average was in school or whether you were able to memorize all the million and one facts about medicine and physiology that you should have, if you're a veterinarian or a veterinary technician. But they can tell that you care about their pets and that you are willing to spend the time to listen to their concerns and answer all their questions. They also appreciate the time and effort you spend to explain a difficult or challenging case.

No matter how much people love their pets and want to take care of them, they often do the wrong things because they are acting on bad information. You have to find a way to counteract all the myths and misconceptions they are getting from their neighbors, friends, and relatives, not to mention the guy at the pet store and the groomer down the street. If you explain their pets' conditions clearly, they won't go to other sources that are misleading, and they won't forgo needed care because they didn't understand why it was important.

As a rule, try not to make decisions for your clients about what care their pets receive. Allow them to make the decision, but make sure it is based on good, up-to-date information and their own preferences.

Clients don't come into your hospital knowing all about pet care. They must be shown how to be good pet owners and what to do to care for their pets. If you and your team aren't teaching them about good pet care, who will? Educating your clients, by talking to them, giving them handouts, and so on, is not optional—it is essential.

When you are part of a veterinary practice team, it is equally important for you to teach each other, especially when someone is new to the job. Your hospital's employees can function well together as a health-care team only when all get the training and mentoring they need to be good, productive employees.

15. Be an Advocate for the Pet

Your patients can't speak for themselves. Even when you do your best to teach pet owners, they don't always understand what their pets need to stay healthy and happy. They may not understand the risks and benefits of procedures, and they may hear false or misleading things from television, relatives, neighbors and friends, trainers, pet store employees, groomers and breeders, or the Internet. They often don't understand the language or concepts of science and medicine. Your job is to stand firm for the needs of the pet, to say, "This is what you need to do for Fluffy today." You must explain the needs of the patient to the owner.

As discussed in point 14 above ("Think of Yourself as a Teacher"), it is the owners' job to decide what level of care they want and can afford. It is your job not only to teach the clients but to speak for the pets.

Whenever possible, it may help to offer two "yes" options to customers rather than a "yes" option and a "no" option. For example, when a client calls and says his or her pet is sick, and you know the pet needs to be seen, you could say, "Oh, that sounds serious. Would you like to bring Buffy in this morning or this afternoon?" This is much more positive and proactive than saying, "Would you like to bring Buffy in for an exam?" Offering two "yes" options suggests to the client that you are confident, positive, and in control. Offering just a "yes" and a "no" sends the message that whatever you are offering isn't really necessary.

Clients often want to know what you would do if it were your pet. Most veterinary team members take excellent care of their own pets. Why would you offer someone else's pet any less than you would offer to your own?

16. Be Patient and Keep Trying

You wouldn't try to sell clients every service you offer on the first visit. Likewise, you should not try to teach them everything about puppy care at the first exam. Start by determining a client's level of knowledge and understanding about pet care and build gradually from there. Bit by bit, the client will absorb more information and act on it. You won't be able to reach every client, nor will your efforts get every patient the best care. But you will sure be further ahead than if you never tried at all.

You also won't get every speech or presentation right. You won't deal well with every client, nor will every customer purchase everything you recommend. Some days you'll blow your presentation entirely or a client will stare at you with an utter lack of comprehension. Don't give up.

You know what's cool about being a human being? You're in charge of yourself! Unlike pets, you get to decide every day what to eat, how much exercise to get, where to go, and what to do every day. It's your choice to be a little better every day or to stay the same, to help coworkers or to ignore them, to wow your clients or to treat them poorly.

Great veterinary team members didn't get there by being the best or smartest in school. They got there by learning to communicate knowledge and skills to others and by getting a little better every day. Set some goals. Read a little, attend a seminar, ask your boss or coworkers for help and guidance, push and stretch yourself to improve. How could you have explained a little better to Ms. Brown why her dog needed a dental cleaning? How could you be a little more effective when talking to phone shoppers? Why was that estimate for Cookie's surgery so far off? Think carefully about your job and your effectiveness as a veterinary employee. Where do you think you are today? Where do you want to be tomorrow?

TWO KINDS OF EDUCATING, FOUR STEPS TO FOLLOW

There are two basic types of client education that veterinary practice team members do every day: educating about diseases and educating about preventive care. Educating about the treatment of diseases and problems is usually done by the doctors. Clients may be stressed or worried in these situations, so we need to be empathetic and caring. Compliance may be critical if the pet is ill, and decisions may need to be made quickly.

Educating clients about wellness and preventive care, however, is often done by the entire team. Clients may be bored or distracted during these talks, so we need to be entertaining as well as informative, and we have more time than we do when educating clients in crisis situations. Both types of education require communication skills, but educating clients about problems or disease may require more medical knowledge.

When it comes to wellness care, especially, we are all teachers. Veterinarians talk to clients about wellness, of course, but so does almost everyone else in the hospital. Since this book was written for the entire team, the majority of the book focuses more on the wellness part of client education; you can also refer to books specifically on communication, and veterinary communication in particular. (See the Resources listed at the end of this section.) I want to spend a little time here on how to talk about diseases and problems, since that can be particularly challenging.

When the pet is sick or needs a major procedure, it's more likely that the doctor or a skilled technician will be speaking to the client about diagnosing or treating the problem. Getting a history of the pet's problem, though, often involves multiple team members. The CRS may need to get a history in order to figure out how urgent the problem is and how soon the patient needs to come in, and he or she may need to explain to the client what to do in the meantime. For example, the CRS may have to tell the client to withhold food from a vomiting patient or explain how to transport an injured pet to the hospital. Once the client and pet arrive, additional history notes may be taken by a technician or assistant in the exam room.

These steps are critical in the process of diagnosis and treatment and eventually will help to determine what we are educating clients about and how. Good communication involves listening to and filtering information, not just delivering it. Furthermore, how we go about these tasks will affect how the clients perceive us and how they will accept and act on the information we give them later on.

There are four parts to discussing a disease problem with a client. These are as follows:

1. **Engage**—Your goal is to get a story, not an answer, at this stage. The search is for meaning, not so much for facts, although those are important, too.
2. **Empathize**—The client cares and is worried about the pet. We have to demonstrate that we understand this.
3. **Educate**—The client should understand the diagnosis, the treatment plan, and the options that are presented.
4. **Enlist**—Involve the client in planning for the pet's care and get buy-in, or the owner will not actually comply with the doctor's recommendations.

Let's look at each of these steps in more detail.

ENGAGE

In human medicine, 80 percent of the diagnostic rule-outs come from what the patient tells the doctor—the history and symptoms (Peterson et al. 1992). This is equally true in veterinary medicine. For instance, knowing the pet had blood and mucous in the diarrhea means the doctor needs to focus on diseases that affect the colon. Knowing the vomit looked like phlegm and mucous tells us the problem may be a throat infection vs. a stomach problem. Getting good information is just as important as doing a thorough physical exam or ordering the right lab tests. Good ways to go about this are outlined in the "Questioning Your Clients" section of this book.

EMPATHIZE

Clients want to feel heard and understood. Be a mirror reflecting the speaker: Repeat some of the words you have heard and summarize what you think the owner is telling you. Your nonverbal communication should be attentive, nonjudgmental, and open. Use caring phrases, such as "I know you don't want him to suffer anymore," or "You've made the right choice for you and your family." Acknowledge their feelings with phrases like "You look worried" and "You seem to be hesitating."

Many times the owner is fretting about something to do with the pet's care based on prior personal experiences with veterinary or human health care. Someone whose family member was treated or died from a similar disease, or who had similar symptoms, often leaps to the wrong conclusions. His or her mind may be spinning so fast he or she can't hear what you are saying. If you know the client well enough, you may be able to anticipate some of this. Often what the client thinks is going on or is important is far from the truth, so you have to be careful that you understand exactly what the client is thinking so you can make course corrections.

Clients often perceive that we judge them. They worry that we think they have been bad pet owners or are incompetent or are making wrong decisions. They are afraid they may appear stupid if they ask questions or admit they don't understand something. That's why they don't tell us things we need to know, such as that they haven't actually been able to give their cat the pills.

You *always* need to keep this in mind when hard decisions need to be made—the client is not only worried about the pet, she's worried about what you think of her. Even if the client doesn't tell you she feels this way, you need to say things like "Whatever you decide, you will have made a good decision."

You may want to eliminate physical barriers—like the exam table—between you and the client. Sit next to a stressed client rather than facing him or her head on. He or she will feel as if you are an ally and relax, and may be more open about concerns.

Educate

When explaining a disease process or treatment plan, frame your questions to a client very carefully. People learn best by talking about what they've learned, so having them explain the new information back to you will help them to remember it better. You must also give them chances to ask questions, and at the same time attempt to empathize with how they are doing, using the "mirroring" technique described above. Try using some of the following phrases:

"Diabetes is a tough disease to explain and I've given you a lot of information. What didn't I explain well enough?"

"Is what I am saying making sense to you? Am I talking too fast?"

"You will need to explain this to your spouse. Let's go over it again so you feel comfortable explaining it to him when you get home."

"This is complex; a lot of people don't get it all the first time."

"You look like you're feeling overwhelmed."

Slow down and allow time for the client to process the information. Provide it in chunks, then stop and check for understanding:

"Do you have questions about the insulin administration before I move on to talk about diet and a feeding schedule?"

"I've gone over quite a bit with you—it may be hard to take it in all at once. Before I continue, what questions do you have so far about your pet's surgery?"

Do the same after you talk about the aftercare, and again when you discuss rehab.

Be very specific with your recommendations. For example, don't say, "Take Fido on short walks." Specify five minutes or two blocks. Don't say, "Three times a day." Say, "Every eight hours." "Once daily" is not the same as "one pill daily," but in the client's mind it may be!

According to the Institute of Medicine, 42 percent of public hospital patients in one study could not understand medication directions to "give on an empty stomach." Only half of American adults are medically literate, and 60 percent of adults over age 60 have inadequate or marginal health-care literacy skills (Institute of Medicine 2004). As patients, people who do not have good health literacy are less likely to make use of screening tests such as mammograms than patients who do. They also present to doctors later in a disease process, are hospitalized more often, and are much less likely to take medications. People do not trust that which they do not understand—and if that is what they do when it comes to their own health, it certainly affects how they deal with the health of their pets.

Ninety million Americans have difficulty reading a prescription label, following simple instructions, or understanding a diagnosis. As medicine becomes more complex each year, these problems will only get worse. In addition, people are often embarrassed to admit they don't understand, so they nod their head yes, and then go home and fail to comply. Many of the smiling faces that exit through our doors leave having no idea what we just said. Fecal sample? What's that? Cruciate what? What is a ligament? Is glucose the same as sugar?

Even intelligent, well-educated adults become confused when dealing with a lot of information outside their field of expertise. Our clients are often distracted, stressed, or worried about their pet, making the challenge even greater. If the client seems to be lost in a fog, it's your job to notice that, and either start over or save some information for next time.

Finally, if we don't believe the messenger, we won't believe the message. It's all about credibility. This is why clients often believe the practice owner but not the new associate doctor. The older or more experienced you appear to be, the more credible you are to the client. The more confident and composed your body language, and the more questions you can answer, the more believable you will be. Getting inside the client's mind and showing empathy for his or her fears and frustrations can help overcome some of this—it makes you look very smart.

ENLIST

Compliance is defined as "yielding to pressure, demand, or coercion." It is when a client does what we say because we are experts giving orders—for example, "You need to give these heartworm pills."

Adherence is "agreeing to join, being consistent or in accord." This occurs when we say, "I'd like to discuss with you how to prevent heartworm disease. Is that okay?" and the client agrees. This way of phrasing your recommendations enlists the client as an equal instead of dictating as if he or she were inferior.

Your goal should be for clients to adhere to your recommendations, not just comply with them. There are several ways to accomplish this.

For example, to assess whether a client will opt for the surgery you are recommending, you can ask, "How convinced are you that this surgery will help Rusty?" or, "On a scale of 1 to 10, how confident are you that you can give Frisky the medicine?" If the answer is a 5 or 6, you didn't convince the client! Regroup and go at it again or from another angle.

Believe body language over words. If you ask the client, "Will you be able to give the medication?" and he says yes but his body language or tone is hesitant, he probably won't give it. If that is the case, you can take more time to find out what is keeping the client from feeling comfortable with administering the medication.

Again, clients don't want to admit they didn't understand or cannot do something. They also don't understand the consequences of not following your directions unless you tell them what they are. Explain consequences, and plan for mistakes:

"If you don't give the pain medication, Frisky won't cry out, but that doesn't mean he's not in pain."

"If you miss a dose of insulin, here's what you need to do . . ."

"If you forget to give a heartworm pill on the first, give it as soon as you remember, then resume your once-a-month schedule."

Everything you explain should also be sent home in writing. Clients remember less than 20 percent of what they hear in the exam room (Kolb 1984). It is critical that they be able to refer back to what you send home with them, or mistakes are almost guaranteed to happen. You should be sending home clear explanations of diseases and problems, clear descriptions of the treatments needed, and clear instructions for what you want clients to do.

Last, follow up with your clients. It is critically important that we call the pet owner back or schedule the recheck to make sure we are doing all we can to ensure the treatment needs of the pet are being met. These same sorts of questions are vital to ensuring that we catch nonadherence early and come up with solutions to problems or complications. These communication principles are important for all kinds of discussions with clients, but they are especially important for discussions about medical problems.

RESOURCES

American Animal Hospital Association. 2003. *The Path to High-Quality Care*. Lakewood, CO: AAHA Press.

Antech Diagnostics Online, www.antechdiagnostics.com.

Bonvicini, Kathleen A., and Karen K. Cornell. 2008. "Are Clients Truly Informed? Communication Tools and Risk Reduction." *Compendium* 30, no. 11 (November): 572–578, https://secure.vlsstore.com/ME2/Audiences/dirmod.asp?sid=F0E2AE6B0B7E437588DFCF8A9FCA8CAC&nm=CE+Programs&type=Publishing&mod=Publications%3A%3AArticle&mid=8F3A7027421841978F18BE895F87F791&AudID=BE924B06C44442DE9033CA13B621B284&tier=4&id=6DB9367678D144EC836E89F5EB08554C. This is an excellent article on communication skills and teaches the "ask-tell-ask" and "chunk-and-check" techniques for delivering in-depth medical information to clients.

Boss, Nan. 2003. *The Client Education Notebook: Customized Client Education Materials to Use in Your Own Practice*. Lincoln, NE: AVLS-PetCom. Volume 1 includes handout sets for puppies, kittens, adult cats and dogs, and senior cats and dogs. These materials focus on wellness and preventive care. They are provided in Microsoft Word format on CD so that you can customize them to your practice. Volume 2 contains medication information sheets and a variety of client handouts on topics not covered elsewhere. Some are about symptoms that need to be worked up (vs. diseases or diagnoses). Others are on fun behavior topics such as the role of play in dog training—focusing not on a behavior problem but on how pet owners can nurture positive relationships with their dogs.

Career Track, www.CareerTrack.com. Click on "Seminars" to see the schedule of seminars being offered in or near your city. There are a number of companies like Career Track that give seminars on business topics in cities across the United States. Veterinary hospitals aren't that different from other businesses, since we deal with customer service, management, and human resource issues like any other type of company. Don't limit yourself to veterinary-specific training programs. See also Pryor.com and Skillpath.com listed below.

Carnegie, Dale. 1952. *How to Win Friends and Influence People*. Englewood Cliffs, NJ: Prentice Hall. This was the very first book I ever read on communications and people skills and it remains one of the best. See the Dale Carnegie Training website, www.dalecarnegie.com/, for other helpful materials. If you are interested in courses on public speaking, look for a Dale Carnegie course offered in your community. If you are looking for information on other business topics, click on "search topics."

Downing, Robin. 2003. *Cornerstones of Compliance*. Guelph, Ontario: Lifelearn. See www.lifelearn.com/c4/4019.html. These interactive team training materials by Dr. Robin Downing are part of Lifelearn's Compliance Series, which includes interactive CDs on *Dental Compliance, Nutritional Compliance, Parasite Management/Zoonotic Disease Management Compliance*, and *Vaccination Compliance*. Lifelearn also sells client handout sets for cats, dogs, exotics, oncology, and many other topics.

Fred Pryor Seminars, www.Pryor.com. Fred Pryor Seminars and Career Track (listed above) are both part of PARK University Enterprises. Click on "Seminars" for seminars being offered in your area.

Kelly, Christine Kuehn. 2001. "Good Diagnostic Skills Should Begin at the Bedside: Improving Physical Exams and History-Taking Can Help You Become More Efficient and Compassionate." ACP Internist, www.acpinternist.org/archives/2001/02/diagnostics.htm. Reprinted from the *ACP-ASIM Observer*, February 2001.

Lagoni, Laurel, and Dana Durrance. 2010. *Connecting with Clients: Practical Communication Techniques for 15 Common Situations*, 2nd ed. Lakewood, CO: AAHA Press.

Shula, Don, and Ken Blanchard. 1995. *Everyone's a Coach*. New York: Harper Business Press.

SkillPath Seminars, www.SkillPath.com. Click on "View Our Seminars" and look at those listed under "Customer Service," "Management & Supervisory," or "Personal Development & Communication."

Smith, Carin. 2009. *Client Satisfaction Pays: Quality Service for Practice Success*, 2nd ed. Lakewood, CO: AAHA Press.

Soares, Cecilia J. 1999. *One Client at a Time: Communicating the Value of Your Services*. Lakewood, CO: AAHA Press. DVD and workbook.

Tilley, Larry P., and Francis W.K. Smith Jr. 2008. *Blackwell's Five-Minute Veterinary Consult: Canine and Feline*, 4th ed. New York: Blackwell. This book comes with a great set of client handouts on CD, covering many disease topics.

Veterinary Information Network, www.veterinarypartner.com. This client website contains some helpful client handouts on uncommon disease problems in pets.

APPOINTMENTS

Nothing is more important to the smooth operation of a veterinary practice than optimal scheduling. Too many appointments, and clients may feel rushed. Over time, doctors and team members may begin to feel tense and cranky, and patients may not receive the best possible care. Too few appointments, and the team can get bored and edgy. The clinic's finances may also suffer. Either way, haphazard scheduling impairs the efficiency and effectiveness of the veterinary team.

How you make appointments affects how the client perceives your customer service and your practice. A friendly voice on the telephone gives the client a good impression, and a smiling face behind the desk when the client comes in preserves that good impression. Do your best to arrange a time convenient for the client, and give every patient a high level of care. At the same time, the patient's and client's needs must be balanced with the needs of the team. Care can be compromised if the team is stressed or tired, feels hurried, or has missed lunch three days in a row. Keep the appointment book full but not overbooked.

When scheduling an appointment, you must first know what the appointment is for. Sick animals need to be seen much sooner than those needing routine vaccinations. If the matter is urgent, you might say, "That sounds serious. I'm sure the doctor will want to see her today." Offer the next two available times, or suggest that the pet be admitted for in-hospital care. You can ask, "Will you be able to make it here by 5:30?" If the client seems worried, you could say, "I'm sure we can get Smokey an appointment today, Mr. Bartel." Use the word "admitted" when discussing a hospital stay. To the client, calling it a "drop-off" sounds like taking dirty laundry to the cleaners instead of bringing in a treasured pet for health care.

Some multidoctor practices believe in sharing clients equally so that clients will feel comfortable with each practitioner. Others prefer that each doctor develop his or her own clientele. You might need to ask which doctor the client prefers, depending on your practice's philosophy.

When it is a routine visit, you should have the patient's information before you so that you can see what might be needed at this visit. You could say something like, "I'm so glad you called. It looks like Mickey's vaccinations are a little overdue." To begin the scheduling, you could add, "What is a convenient day and time for you?" Always keep your questions simple, with no more than two options. If a client relations specialist hurriedly gives the client a list of times ("Do you want the 1:00, 2:15, 3:45, 4:30, 5:15, or 5:45?"), the client will be totally confused. Instead, ask if the client prefers morning or afternoon and then offer two time slots. Check the patient's status quickly to see what other matters need to be addressed at this appointment, and let the client know if there is a particular procedure to be taken care of. For example: "It looks like Bronco is due for his heartworm test, too, Ms. Smith. Would you like to schedule that as well?" Always restate the appointment date and time at the end of the phone call to avoid misunderstandings.

If the client is new, you might want to state the clinic's financial policies. For example, "All payments are due at time of service. We take cash, checks, Visa, and MasterCard." This saves a hassle when the client stands at the checkout counter and says, "Can't you bill me?" Don't let payment information be the last thing you say before you hang up, however. Go on to ask, "Do you know where we are located?" or say, "We look forward to meeting you and Barney this afternoon."

Clients are more likely to arrive on time if you state clearly how much time you have allowed for them. For instance, "All right, Ms. Foster, we have 20 minutes blocked off for you to see Dr. Simons, beginning at 9:40. We look forward to seeing you then." If the appointment is scheduled with a technician and not the doctor, be sure the client understands this. You might say, "Heartworm testing is usually done by our technician. Does Fluffy have any health problems that need to be seen by the doctor?"

Consider arranging your scheduling times to avoid round numbers. Clients are more likely to be on time if the appointment is made for an uneven number, such as 4:55 rather than 5:00. This makes the time seem more precise and important.

Be sure you have blocked off enough time for the client. For clients who love to talk, you may need to allow an extra 10 minutes so you don't get behind when they want to chat. A new client will probably need 10 extra minutes before the appointment to fill out paperwork. Some computer programs will tell you how much time to allow for each type of appointment. If your software doesn't do this, you may want to put together a master chart for the entire front-office team.

Euthanasia appointments should be handled with special care. Try to schedule them during a slow time or at the end of an appointment block so the client doesn't have to encounter other people in the waiting room. Be sure everyone knows that a euthanasia is scheduled. Don't let team members hang around chatting or laughing where the distraught client can hear or see them.

Offer a little extra information or help to every customer. Perhaps you could suggest an evening appointment, or an overnight stay, for a client whose request for a Saturday appointment can't be filled. Maybe a technician could call back to discuss the behavior problem a client is having with his or her puppy. Offer to give clients an estimate for the services they are requesting.

Schedule another appointment for a client who calls to cancel one. Don't forget to ask for stool samples if testing is needed. Last, always thank the client for calling.

It is impossible to diagnose a disease over the phone. If the pet is sick, get the patient into the hospital. Offer two "yes" questions. For example, if the client says, "My dog has been coughing for three days. What should I do?" your answer is, "You were right to call us. This is the kind of case the doctor needs to see. Would you like to come in this morning or this afternoon?" Wording it this way gives the client two ways to say, "Yes, I want to bring my dog in," and no way to refuse. You have given the owner positive reinforcement, as well as sounding knowledgeable and efficient. Do not give the option of not bringing the pet in if it needs to be seen.

Avoid offering advice on care or treatment over the phone. If you misinterpret the situation and offer the wrong care, the pet won't get better and may get worse. The owner will be displeased and so will the doctor. If the client says, "Isn't there something I could do for him at home?" say, "I'm sure there will be after the doctor has examined him."

You may need to repeat yourself a few times before the owner gets the message, but most clients do want to have their pet taken care of. They will eventually let you schedule an appointment for them. Clients want to be reassured that they weren't foolish to have called. They also may be anxious about bringing the pet in. They may know he or she is frightened of the hospital, or they could be worried about the cost of care or about having to miss work or postpone other plans. Be sensitive to the client's concerns and try to resolve them. In sales lingo, this is called "comforting the sale." The client wants to feel good about his or her decision to bring the pet in, so you must provide reassurance.

Your goal is to make the client feel good, important, and clever. Make the client glad to have picked up the phone to call you.

BEHAVIOR AND TRAINING

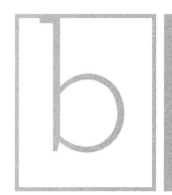

A leading cause of death in dogs is euthanasia for behavior problems. Many of these pets have had little or no training and are exhibiting normal animal behaviors that their owners simply don't know how to handle.

Excessive barking or chewing, separation anxiety, and many other problem behaviors are rampant. As lifestyles get busier and busier, more and more pets are spending large amounts of time home alone and getting into trouble. Some of these behaviors are mere annoyances, while others cause suffering for the pet. Behavior problems in pets can also cause human suffering. About 800,000 Americans seek medical attention for dog bites each year, according to the Centers for Disease Control and Prevention. Of those, 386,000 require treatment in an emergency department.

About half of all dog bites are to children, especially those between the ages of five and nine. Approximately 50 percent of the children bitten are under age 12. In fact, almost all children 12 years of age or older have been bitten at least once by a dog (CDC 2009). This is a serious problem. Because of their size, children are more likely to be bitten in the face than adults, and thus more likely to require medical attention.

Punishment methods of training have been shown to worsen aggression in pets. The majority of dogs presented to behavior specialists for problem aggression have been trained by their owners at home using punishment methods (Herron et al. 2009). When owners are given good information about how to train their pets at the beginning, they are more likely to use the appropriate methods.

An interesting study done in 2007 explored gender differences as well as the effect of reward versus punishment in training dogs. This research showed that the majority of men (93 percent) punished and controlled their dogs more and rewarded them less. As a result, their dogs had more training problems. The majority of women (69.9 percent) rewarded the dogs more, punished them less, and used moderate control. Their dogs were more obedient and had fewer behavior problems (Eskeland et al. 2007).

These sobering statistics tell us there is a need for education of both adults and children about animal handling. Teaching people how to interact with animals and how to choose the right pet should be a goal for every veterinary hospital. How can you help?

One way is to let clients and potential clients know that information is available on choosing the right pet, training the pet, and caring for it. You can help to teach proper pet-training techniques. You can also aid parents in teaching their children about animal handling. Much of this teaching can be done with the use of books, handouts, videos, and other resources that you share with families. Make sure you have good educational materials available in your office. The American Animal Hospital Association has an activity book called *Pets' Playground: Playing Safe in a Dog-and-Cat World* that teaches children how to properly care for pets and be safe around them. You can also recommend reliable online sources of information.

Give clients all the information they can handle on any pet breed or species they are interested in. Make it known through newsletters, your website, and word of mouth that team members at your clinic are available to discuss new pet purchases. Giving tours of your clinic and presentations to grade school children are both great ways to spread the word about good pet care and living compatibly with pets. You can make presentations at your local humane society or high school career day, or you can have a booth at festivals and provide handouts. Perhaps the local newspaper would be open to printing articles written by one of the veterinarians or technicians at your practice. If so, everyone on the team might have good ideas for topics to cover—and pet behavior issues would certainly be of interest to readers.

> **Think of yourself as a teacher.**

When you are interacting with clients one on one, demonstrate good techniques with their pets. Use visits to your practice to teach children how to care for their pets as well as how to avoid getting hurt by strange animals. Children will watch closely to see how others interact with pets. If adults show respect for a pet's feelings and concern for the pet's health and safety, children will learn to do the same. This is also how we acquire the next generation of veterinary clients!

At the end of this section is a handout you can copy and use when you are interacting with children, whether in an exam room or when doing a school talk or practice tour. There are forms and handouts in many sections of this book for you to duplicate and use in your practice (they can also be found on this book's accompanying website, www.aahanet.org/EYC/).

People often acquire pets without understanding the animal's care requirements or natural behaviors. They are sometimes shocked to find out what they have gotten themselves into. Owners need to be educated about behavior to minimize problems that lead to these pets being euthanized or surrendered to shelters.

Teach clients that the more skilled and reward-based the training, the more well adjusted and friendly the dog will be. When a pet is new and the client comes in for its first visit, it's a good opportunity for your team to start this education process. As with children, there are certain ages at which the brains of puppies and kittens are developing in certain ways. You can take advantage of these windows of opportunity to shape their behavior patterns, making them better pets for the rest of their lives. If a puppy or kitten is started off on the right foot, he or she will be a better companion for the next 10 to 15 years. You can reinforce this information often in later visits and provide handouts and training about any specific behavior issues. Continue to model good interaction with the pet.

> **Be an advocate for the pet.**

Team members can show clients how to socialize and handle their pets. This includes handling their feet, ears, and mouth to prepare them for grooming and health-care activities. Encourage owners to work with their pets every day, especially when they are young. If they are taught to submit to these things early in life, pets will allow pilling, nail trimming, ear cleaning, and other treatments quietly and calmly. You must demonstrate these techniques and then watch the client do them, too.

The team can encourage clients to provide lots of social interaction for their pets. Studies show that the more people a six-week-old kitten interacts with, the more social it will be all its life and the more it will interact with its owners. We've all seen feral cats that received little, if any, handling or exposure to people when they were young. Fear of unfamiliar things is an adaptive trait in the wild, and it is a dominant gene, so it is difficult to get rid of by breeding. Fear is diminished through early and frequent contact with people. Feral cats never learn to like people or bond with them very well and tend to be either shy or aggressive. Puppies, too, need lots of exposure to new people, other pets, and children at a young age.

> *Fear of unfamiliar things is an adaptive trait in the wild, and it is a dominant gene, so it is difficult to get rid of by breeding.*

If your clinic offers behavior counseling, be sure pet owners are told about this opportunity more than once. Ask your clients to call if they have questions or problems with any aspect of their pets' behavior, including barking, biting, digging, and chewing. Tell cat owners to call immediately if they notice litter-box avoidance or spraying. Give people these specific examples, because they don't always know what is meant by "behavior problems." Talk about behavior issues at every puppy and kitten visit. With every annual exam, ask owners if problems exist. If you don't tell them behavior counseling is available, clients will assume you can't help them with these problems.

Repetition is key!

If you don't have a trainer or someone interested in behavior at your hospital, it is imperative that you have someone to whom you can refer your clients when these issues arise. Clients may be desperate or very frustrated by the time they finally call for help, especially when it comes to serious behavior issues. Their needs must be addressed quickly and thoroughly. The more team members can help with basic behavior recommendations the better, and in my hospital it's a requirement for everyone to do some reading and watch DVDs on behavior, restraint, and aggression. Being an expert in behavior problems takes years of study, but everyone on the practice team should know at least the basics.

> **The entire team must be great communicators!**

There are a lot of great tools available nowadays that you can teach clients about, too. Head halters, harnesses, indestructible or rubber toys, Scat mats, indoor invisible fence systems, pheromone products, citronella collars—all these things can help clients to solve or prevent simple behavior problems. If your clinic sells some of these items, every team member should learn about them so that they can be recommended as needed. Team members should know how to give instructions on their use as well.

Most of the knowledge base in animal behavior has developed in the past 25 years. Although dogs, cats, and people have lived together for thousands of years, relatively few formal behavior studies were done until recently. As a result, clients have been exposed to a lot of misinformation and many old wives' tales. These include the old "rub his nose in it" or "swat him with a rolled-up newspaper" theories, the "she pees on the living room rug because she's mad at me" theory, and the "prong collars are the only way to get your dog to listen" theory.

Holding puppy- and kitten-training sessions at your clinic is a great way to teach clients good pet care, bond them to the practice, and bring in a little extra income as well. *First Steps with Puppies and Kittens: A Practice-Team Approach to Behavior,* by Linda M. White, teaches veterinary teams how to hold puppy and kitten classes and consultations.

Team members also need to know that not all behavior problems result from bad training. It is a mistake to assume that medical and behavior problems are always two separate issues. They aren't. Brain tumors and low thyroid levels can cause aggression in dogs, as can any painful condition, such as arthritis. Bladder infections can cause cats to spray. In fact, socialization begins in the

> **Think of yourself as a teacher.**

womb. Stress on the mother leads to changes in hormone levels, which lead to changes in the puppies. This may be true for cats as well. Moreover, even when the problem is truly behavioral, a physical exam is needed. To use behavior-modifying drugs, the doctor must have current blood work to assess liver and kidney function. In other words, no matter what the problem is, the veterinarian will want to do a physical exam and blood, urine, and/or stool testing. Never refer a client to a trainer or offer behavioral advice unless the pet has been examined.

Socialization begins in the womb. Stress on the mother leads to changes in hormone levels, which lead to changes in the puppies. This may be true for cats as well.

Until a few years ago, information on treating animals with behavior-modifying drugs was limited. Today, many disorders, from carsickness to carpet soiling, can be treated with a combination of behavior training and drug treatments. It all starts with the efforts of your team to let clients know that help and treatment are available for the asking.

RESOURCES

Advanstar Communications. 2007. *Canine Behavior Problems: A Four-Step Approach.* Woodland Hills, CA: Advanstar. This publication is a 16-page compilation of behavior articles focusing on implementation of behavioral programs in a practice situation.

Alley Cat Allies, www.alleycat.org.

American Animal Hospital Association. 2008. "Doggie Manners." Lakewood, CO: AAHA Press. This is a two-sided activity sheet that teaches bite-safety tips. AAHA Press also carries a Pet Behavior Brochure series of pamphlets that provide information and advice about many common behavioral problems.

American Association of Feline Practitioners, www.catvets.com. The AAFP published its Feline Behavior Guidelines in 2004, available online at www.catvets.com/professionals/guidelines/publications/?Id=177. The association also has a position statement from 2009 entitled "Respectful Handling of Cats to Prevent Fear and Pain," online at www.

catvets.com/uploads/PDF/Nov2009HandlingCats.pdf. "Feline Handling Techniques" will be released in 2011. The website includes many other articles as well that would be useful for client education. See also "Creating a Cat Friendly Practice," at www.fabcats.org/catfriendlypractice/guides.html.

American Veterinary Society of Animal Behavior, www.avsabonline.org. The website has information on many behavioral topics as well as position statements. See "Guidelines on the Use of Punishment for Dealing with Behavior Problems in Animals," www.avsabonline.org/avsabonline/images/stories/punishment%20guidelines-aversives%20effects-definitions.pdf.

Animal Behavior Resources, Inc., abrionline.org. This website offers lists of behavior articles and abstracts.

Centers for Disease Control and Prevention, www.cdc.gov. Look under the "Injury, Violence & Safety" menu for the topic "Dog Bites," or under the "Safety at Home, School or Work" menu for the topic "Pet/Animal Safety."

Chin, Amanda. 2009. *Pets' Playground: Playing Safe in a Dog-and-Cat World*. Lakewood, CO: AAHA Press. This is a 100-page activity book that teaches children pet-safety techniques and helps them understand dog and cat behavior.

Dogwise, www.dogwise.com. Dogwise carries many books on behavior, including client-education booklets by Sarah Whitehead. Titles include *Gentle Hands Off Dog Training*, *Adolescent Dog Survival Guide*, *Dogs Are from Neptune*, *Visiting the Dog Park*, and many others.

DVM360, www.dvm360.com. This site lists several behavior tools. Under the "Business Center" menu, choose "Patient Care Forms." Look for "Pre-adoption Counseling Resources," "Behavior Questionnaire," "Behavior Assessment Checklist," and "Behavior History Form." Under "Client Handouts" you'll find "Overcoming Common Behavior Problems in Kittens," "Bringing Home Baby: Introducing a Pet to Your New Arrival," "Teaching Your New Puppy the Right Way to Play," "Why Punishment Fails; What Works Better," "Feline Behavior Q & A," "Listen Closely for Clues on Pet Behavior," and "How to Create Low-Stress Veterinary Visits for Cats."

Hunthausen, Wayne. 2010. "7 Steps to a Profitable Behavior Program." *Veterinary Economics*, June 1.

James and Kenneth Publishers, www.jamesandkenneth.com. This publisher offers wonderful books, DVDs, and behavior booklets by Dr. Ian Dunbar, including lots of materials on puppy training and socialization. These are great materials to use in developing puppy classes, especially the *SIRIUS® Puppy Training* DVD and Doctor Dunbar's 2003 *Good Little Dog* book.

Kilcommons, Brian, and Sarah Wilson. 1999. *Paws to Consider: Choosing the Right Dog for You and Your Family*. New York: Warner Books.

McConnell, Patricia B. 1996. *Dog's Best Friend's Beginning Family Dog Training*. Black Earth, WI: Dog's Best Friend. Dog's Best Friend also carries Dr. McConnell's booklets on behavior problems, including separation anxiety, litter-box avoidance, and other topics. These are inexpensive resources that you can sell to clients.

———. 2002. *The Other End of the Leash: Why We Do What We Do Around Dogs*. New York: Ballantine.

Morris Animal Foundation, www.MorrisAnimalFoundation.org. This foundation has established the R. K. Anderson Animal Behavior Research Endowment to prevent the leading cause of death in young dogs. The endowment will fund research targeting prevention and improvement of pet behavior problems.

Overall, Karen L. 1997. *Clinical Behavioral Medicine for Small Animals*. Oxford, UK: Mosby Year Book. This book contains a pullout section of handouts to reproduce for clients, as well as comprehensive information on behavior. A more recent book by Dr. Overall is *Handbook of Small Animal Behavioral Medicine*, published by Saunders in 2007.

Premier Pet Products, www.premier.com. This company offers the Gentle Leader head halter collar and Gentle Spray no-bark collars. These are humane and effective tools to help with behavior problems in dogs, including jumping, pulling, barking, and aggression. A little training booklet comes with the collar as well as promotional pamphlets and DVDs. There are often live demonstrations of the Gentle Leader halter at veterinary conferences.

"Puppy Tutors Generate Revenue, Happy Clients." 2007. *Veterinary Economics*, January 1.

"Solving Pet Behavior Problems Is an Entire Veterinary Team Effort." 2008. *Veterinary Economics*, October 1.

Wagner, Marlene. 2007. "Sit! Speak! Educate!!" *Veterinary Economics*, April 1.

Walkowicz, Chris. 1996. *The Perfect Match: A Buyer's Guide to Dogs*. New York: Wiley.

White, Linda M. 2009. *First Steps with Puppies and Kittens: A Practice-Team Approach to Behavior*. Lakewood, CO: AAHA Press.

Wombacher, Mike. 2001. *There's a Baby in the House! Preparing Your Dog for the Arrival of Your Child*. www.doggonegood.org.

Yin, Sophia, behavior4veterinarians.com. Yin's videos, articles, and client handouts are available here.

CHILDREN AND DOGS: LIVING COMPATIBLY

Dogs Like It When You . . .
- Treat them with respect and kindness.
- Approach them from the front.
- Ask their owner's permission before petting.
- Let them sniff you before you begin petting.
- Stand still and quiet when they approach you.
- Let them know you are near by talking softly or whistling and not startling them.

Dogs Do Not Like It When You . . .
- Run past them or turn your back on them and run away. A dog's instinct is to chase and catch fleeing prey.
- Approach them when they are confined or restrained, especially if they do not know you.
- Disturb them while they are sleeping, eating, or guarding something. Dogs naturally guard their food, puppies, and toys. Dogs also protect their owners, as well as any property that belongs to their owners, such as a home, a yard, or their cars.
- Put your hands between them and another dog.
- Put your face too close to theirs.
- Pull anything out of their mouth, such as a bone, toy, or stick.
- Pick up and carry dogs that are not your own.
- Chase or tease them.
- Approach a dog that is injured. Children should be instructed to tell an adult if they see an injured dog.

If Threatened by a Dog . . .
- Remain calm and quiet.
- Try to remain motionless until the dog moves away, then back up slowly until he or she is out of sight. Most dogs will only sniff you, decide you aren't a threat, and walk away.
- Remember that if you fall or are knocked to the ground, you should curl into a ball with your hands over your ears and remain motionless. Try not to scream or roll around.

Handout by the Wisconsin VMA, 2801 Crossroads Drive, Suite 1200, Madison, WI 53718. Phone: 1-608-257-3665.

CANCER

There is nothing that pet owners dread more than a diagnosis of cancer. "The Big C," we sometimes call it. Most clients view cancer in pets as a death sentence, even though that is far from being the case. Because of fear and their experiences and knowledge about cancer care in humans, they often will reflexively decline care before receiving all the facts. Moreover, they usually lack a good understanding about what can be done to prevent cancer.

As a member of the veterinary practice team, you must know some basic information about cancer in companion animals. The doctors are the experts, but as a technician, assistant, or client relations specialist, you will also be interacting with clients who have just heard this diagnosis. They have decisions to make about their pets' treatment and may need additional support. You will need to be prepared to help in ways that you can, while referring them to the doctor for things that require his or her medical training and knowledge.

Dogs and cats become more susceptible to cancer as they age, just as humans do. Cancer, also called *neoplasia*, is the leading cause of death in older dogs. It is the second leading cause of death in older cats (kidney failure being first cause for the feline). About half of all older dogs and one-third of all older cats die of cancer. However, a cancer diagnosis is not always a death sentence. More and more pets who are diagnosed with this disease are now beating it (Rusk and Khanna 2005). Oncology is the fastest-growing veterinary specialty, not only because it's so common but also because there is more and more we can do to treat it.

There are as many types of cancer as there are types of cells in the body, and they can cause a variety of disease symptoms and problems, from lameness to internal bleeding to panting, or even diarrhea. Cancer can sound very complicated when it is discussed in medical journals. In reality, it is not hard to understand what is happening. In cancer, the cells simply multiply when they are not supposed to, forming a lump, invading other tissues, and sometimes spreading through the lymphatic system or the bloodstream to other parts of the body (called *metastasizing*). The symptoms and progress of the disease depend on how large the resulting tumor is, how fast the cancer spreads, and how it affects the systems of the body. Different species and breeds of dogs are prone to different types, although almost any kind of cancer can occur in any breed.

PREVENTION AND EARLY DETECTION

Although most cancers are found in older pets, some types frequently affect younger animals, so no matter what a pet's age, pet owners need to know what to watch for. They should understand that it is important to call whenever they find a lump or notice an unusual symptom. Clients can also learn how they may be able to reduce cancer risk.

> **Repetition is key.**

Repeated messages about cancer treatment when the pet is healthy can also prepare pet owners for any cancer diagnosis that may occur in the future. If clients understand ahead of time that many cancers are not only treatable but curable, they are less likely to panic when they find a lump or you give them that diagnosis.

Many cancers are cured by surgically removing them, so early detection and removal are critical. Pet owners should have all lumps and bumps looked at and should investigate signs of illness promptly, especially in older pets. At the end of this section, a client form is provided that you can copy and use to teach about cancer prevention. It is also provided through AAHA Press at the following website: www.aahanet.org/EYC/

TREATING CANCER

The most common types of cancer in pets are tumors in or just beneath the skin, where they usually can be surgically removed. For other pets, chemotherapy or radiation may be necessary.

Sometimes clients question whether treating a pet for cancer is a "normal" thing to do, especially if they have heard negative comments from friends or family. Some people, even veterinary team members, may ask themselves why we treat cancer in pets. However, many diseases that veterinarians treat cannot be cured, including diabetes, heart disease, and kidney disease, and we treat these disorders without question. Why should cancer be any different? Even in cases where a cure is unlikely, with treatment we can often extend lifespan while preserving an excellent quality of life.

Once the cancer is identified, usually via biopsy, the doctor will discuss treatment options with the client. The prognosis, costs, risks, and benefits of treatment are included in this discussion. The pet owner must then decide whether to have the disease treated. It is imperative that the pet owner receive written information about the pet's disease and be given support for whatever decision he or she eventually makes. As a member of the team, you will likely need to gather handouts, share additional information, and offer emotional support to the client as he or she grieves and weighs options. Below we will discuss this role in greater detail.

If the prognosis is poor, hospice care and good pain management are still options to discuss. Sometimes this is referred to as "pawspice" in veterinary care. Besides keeping the animal as pain-free as possible, this includes management of vomiting and diarrhea and making sure that the pet does not starve or become dehydrated. Whether we are treating the cancer aggressively or providing supportive hospice care, it is a primary goal to minimize suffering in the pet.

MAKING DECISIONS ABOUT TREATMENT

The owner is the one to decide which treatment options to proceed with and when euthanasia is the best option. All owners facing these decisions should be given information about the options, answers to their questions, and an understanding ear. There are three types of people when it comes to making decisions. As a member of the team, your role is to offer support no matter which type of decision-maker you are assisting.

The three types of decision-makers are: (1) those who want to make the decisions themselves; (2) those who want someone to tell them what to do; and (3) those who want to collaborate with a team in making the decision. Your job is to figure out which type of decision-maker is standing before you and deal with him or her accordingly.

When you have clients who fit the first category, it is best to deliver information and then sit back and let them think and decide. Sometimes these clients make a decision even before receiving the information. Unfortunately, this sometimes means they are making an uninformed decision.

It is difficult to communicate options to someone who has already made a decision. As the advocate for the pet, you may have to carefully try to educate clients who seem focused on one choice going in. Listen to the clients' concerns and find out how they came to this decision. Share information in short bursts, and try to involve the entire family. You can say, "This is a very treatable form of cancer and you can take a few days to think it over. Why don't you and Mary read this information over and talk about it? I want to make sure you are making an informed decision and for everyone in the family to be comfortable with your choices." We need to prevent decisions from being made without clients really understanding what the options are. However, once they've made a decision, no matter what it is, it is your job to support it.

With the second type of decision-maker, those who want to be told what to do, you have the opposite challenge. You must be very careful not to make the decision for them, much as they might like you to. It's not your pet or your money on the line—it is theirs—and it has to be their decision, too. This doesn't mean you can't give an opinion, but you have to lay out all the reasonable choices, not just the option you think is best. If you do not present every option, such clients are not making an informed choice, and the decision may not be the best one for them.

What this type of client really wants to know is what you would do if it was your pet. They want to do what is best for the pet, and assume that you will know the answer. For this type of client you can gently ask questions to try to help them work through the decision. What factors will be important to that decision? Cost? Logistics? The personality of the pet? Try to figure out what a client may be wrestling with so you can help. You can ask, "Is the treatment she needs going to cause financial hardship for your family?" Perhaps the client is worried that he or she will be unable to administer treatments or care. Cats, especially, can be very difficult to medicate.

Or perhaps the client feels that visiting the hospital and having repeated blood draws, IV catheters, or other treatments will be too stressful for the pet. Some pets are more affected by stress than others, and usually owners are aware of how their own pets deal with stress. If buying a few months of extra time means the cat will spend those months hiding under the bed because it's so stressed-out, maybe this isn't the right treatment plan in this case. On the other hand, maybe we need to try some creative solutions for the stress reactions. You can ask, "How do you think Herbie will handle the stress of coming to the hospital weekly?"

There might also be family issues, such as a family member who has anxiety issues or is sensitive to change. Or there could be children in the household who are close to the pet. Allow the client to raise these issues without others overhearing so that he or she can "think out loud" about them with someone who is a good listener. When children are involved, encourage the client to involve them in the decision making. This can be difficult, but it is better than having the children feel left out.

Be sure the pet owner knows what kinds of complications may arise. Ask, "Will you still feel okay with this decision if he doesn't do well?" "Would it help you to know that you tried everything you could, or do you think you might regret the effort?" Some people find making decisions very difficult under the best of circumstances, much less when it's life or death. The more information you have, the more you can help, though in the end the choice has to be theirs.

> **Be an advocate for the pet.**

The last group of decision-makers, those who tend to collaborate as a team, want you to give them information and then want to discuss their options and choices with you to come to a decision. This is usually the most satisfying group to work with. If you are lucky, at least one member of the family is in this group.

The most difficult part of negotiating treatment for a serious medical problem is when there are two or more family members involved who think and decide in totally different ways and come to different conclusions. There's nothing more miserable than having one spouse completely unable to let go and the other wanting immediate euthanasia. If we aren't trained to be teachers, we certainly aren't trained to be psychologists! Patience, honesty, and empathy are your best tools in these situations.

If you aren't sure which type of personality you are dealing with, ask. "Do you want me to just give you information or do you want me to actively participate in your decision?" "How comfortable are you with making your choice based on what we've laid out?" Try hard not to give the client a recitation of dry statistics. Instead, share experiences that might be helpful, or paint a picture that makes it easier for the client to grasp the situation.

Part of your job will be as a "mythbuster" to dispel preconceived ideas about cancer. Most people understandably assume that treatments for animals are similar to treatments for people. However, this is not the case. Most people think that chemotherapy, for example, will cause the pet to feel miserable all the time, or lose all its hair. Although the drugs used to treat cancer in pets are the same as those used for people, veterinarians generally use lower doses and fewer drugs at a time, which minimizes adverse effects. Fewer than one-third of animal cancer patients experience unpleasant side effects, and 5 percent or less experience a severe side effect. Should unpleasant side effects occur, dosages can be reduced, different medications can be substituted, or additional medications can be dispensed to decrease them.

Most dogs experience little or no hair loss, though some do lose a large amount of hair (usually the nonshedding breeds that need to see a groomer regularly). Cats may lose whiskers and long guard hairs of their coat. This hair loss is not itchy or painful, however, and when it does occur the hair will grow back upon cessation of the chemotherapy.

Radiation is also a treatment modality laden with misconceptions. In pets, radiation is usually used in a local area, not on the whole body. Systemic (i.e., whole-body) side effects are rare in pets, and when they do occur, they are usually associated with the anesthesia, not the radiation itself.

Many clients are concerned that the pet will spend its last weeks or months in the hospital, as human cancer patients often do. However, almost all veterinary chemotherapy treatments are done in an outpatient setting. Furthermore, most protocols involve a series of treatments and then a period of careful observation. Continuous, indefinite chemotherapy is not the norm. Nor is chemotherapy likely to cause issues with toxicity to family members because of urine or stool contamination. Few chemotherapy drugs are excreted for longer than 48 hours. Normal interactions with a pet during the chemo period are not dangerous.

Finally, clients sometimes worry that a pet is too old for treatment. Age is not a disease, however. In fact, most cancer patients at veterinary clinics are older pets, and statistics show that they can benefit from treatment. One doctor told a story about a collie who had a cancerous spleen removed at age 19 and lived to be 22! (Villalobos 2007).

Pets can often live several months or even years longer with medication than without, and their quality of life during that time is often excellent. Be sure that you know what the options and possible outcomes are for a pet before discussing them with a client. There is nothing worse than a client getting confusing or conflicting information. Ultimately, however, whether a pet is a good candidate for chemotherapy will depend on its overall health, not its chronological age.

New cancer treatments are being developed all the time. Cancer vaccines, molecular and gene therapies, nutritional methods, and many new drugs are expanding our therapy choices. New medications for pain and nausea are helping thousands of pets to cope better with cancer and its treatment. Spending the time to teach clients about their options is a good investment.

Although cancer is very common in pets, it is also often very treatable. Many pets live for years after their cancer diagnosis. Since pets are living so much longer nowadays, there is a good chance of any pet developing one or more kinds of cancer in its lifetime. If this happens, we need to carefully discuss the diagnosis and the treatment options with the pet owner so that together we can plan the best treatment for the situation.

RESOURCES

American Association of Feline Practitioners, www.catvets.com. See the AAFP's list of cancer resources at www.catvets.com/search/search.aspx?Search=go&Submit=search&q=cancer.

American Veterinary Medical Association. "Guidelines for Veterinary Hospice Care." www.avma.org/products/hab/hospice.asp.

August, John. 2010. "Feline Pawspice." In *Consultations in Feline Internal Medicine*, vol. 6. New York: W. B. Saunders.

Bergman, Phillip J. 2004. "Chemotherapy Side Effects and How to Prevent or Stop 'Em." From the 2004 American Board of Veterinary Practitioners (ABVP) conference proceedings, available at Veterinary Information Network (VIN), www.vin.com/Members/SearchDB/misc/m05000/m02936.htm. Access to this website requires member registration, but once you are a member you can access many articles on different veterinary topics.

Downing, Robin. 2000. *Pets Living with Cancer*. Lakewood, CO: AAHA Press.

Gaynor, James S., and William W. Muir III, eds. 2008. *Handbook of Veterinary Pain Management*, 2nd ed. St. Louis: Mosby Elsevier. See Chapter 30, "Hospice and Palliative Care," by Tami Shearer.

International Association of Animal Hospice and Palliative Care, www.IAAHPC.org.

Nakaya, Shannon Fujimoto. 2005. *Kindred Spirit, Kindred Care: Making Decisions on Behalf of Our Animal Companions*. Novato, CA: New World Library.

Nikki Hospice Foundation for Pets, www.PetHospice.org.

Oncura partners, www.OncuraPartners.com. This site has useful information for clients about cancer treatment options. Click on "For the Pet Owner" and choose "Cancer Facts."

Villalobos, Alice. 2007. *Canine and Feline Geriatric Oncology: Honoring the Human-Animal Bond*. New York: Blackwell. Dr. Villalobos's "Quality of Life Scale" handout is available at www.dvm360.com. Under the "Business Center" menu, choose "Patient Care Forms." There is also an "Advance Directive" form there.

Withrow, Stephen J., and David M. Vail. 2007. *Withrow and MacEwen's Small Animal Clinical Oncology*, 4th ed. Oxford, UK: W. B. Saunders. See Chapter 16c, "Pawspice: End of Life and Hospice Care."

PREVENTING CANCER

Cancer is common in older pets, but there are several steps you can take while your pet is young to help prevent it. Here is your step-by-step guide to cancer prevention in your dog or cat. Some of the points also apply to rabbits, guinea pigs, and other small mammals. If you have any questions about any of these guidelines, ask your veterinarian for further information.

- **Have your pet spayed or neutered.** The majority of unspayed female dogs and cats will develop mammary tumors (breast cancer) as they get older. Spaying a female pet before her first heat almost completely eliminates this risk. Spaying and neutering are recommended for rabbits and guinea pigs as well as dogs and cats (about 60 percent of unspayed female rabbits die of uterine cancer by age six). Unneutered male dogs are prone to testicular, perianal, and prostate tumors. Neutering a male dog while he is young, or as soon as he is retired from breeding, prevents many problems.

- **Feed your pet a high-quality diet.** It should be rich in antioxidants and fatty acids. These chemicals help protect cells from age-related deterioration, thus reducing the risk of cancer arising from damaged cells. Pets fed premium diets are healthier and live longer.

- **Don't smoke.** Cancer is more likely to occur in cats living in households with a person who smokes than in households without smokers. Smoke is heavier than air, so pets, who spend most of their time lower to the ground, are more at risk and end up taking a lot of secondhand smoke into their lungs. What's more, cats not only inhale the smoke, but when grooming themselves they lick and swallow ash and particulates that settle onto their fur. Most respiratory diseases in pets occur in households with smokers. Smoking is not only dangerous to you but to your pets as well!

- **Keep your pet at a healthy weight.** A study done by Purina showed a longer life expectancy for pets who were kept at a healthy weight than for heavier pets. Instead of suffering from heart disease, diabetes, or high blood pressure, as you would expect (because that's what happens to overweight people), heavier pets are at risk for developing various cancers. Research shows that fat cells produce toxins that damage other cells in the body and increase cancer risk.

- **Check for lumps and bumps and other symptoms.** Report any lumps you find beneath your pet's skin to your veterinarian right away. If you notice blood in the stool or urine, a persistent cough or hoarseness, difficulty swallowing or chewing, or any other change or symptom, you should also call your pet's doctor. Pets should be examined at least once a year. The earlier a tumor is detected, the better the chance of a cure. Don't wait until your pet gets sick.

- **Get regular cancer screening tests for your pet.** Regular blood and urine screening is important because some types of cancer will cause abnormalities in these areas. Radiographs can be taken of the chest and abdomen each year in older pets to detect lesions in the lungs, liver, spleen, or other organs.

- **Limit sun exposure.** Pink-skinned dogs and cats should have limited sun exposure. White cats are especially prone to getting skin cancer on their ears or nose because of sun exposure.
- **Get biopsies when they are recommended.** Lumps and bumps should be checked by cytology or biopsy, both of which allow us to look at cells from the lump under the microscope. This is often as simple as putting a needle into a lump to get a few cells to examine. The procedure can usually tell us if a lump needs to be removed or not. Many cancer cases are cured by surgery to remove the lump.
- **Test cats for feline leukemia and feline immunodeficiency virus.** These viruses can cause cancer. Fortunately, vaccination is now available for both of them. If a cat goes outdoors frequently, it should be vaccinated. All cats should be tested upon adoption or whenever they have a serious illness, and cats that go outdoors should be retested annually.
- **Be informed about vaccination.** Cats can develop cancer at the site of a vaccine injection. Your veterinarian will discuss current vaccine recommendations, which are designed to decrease the risk, but you'll also want to notify your pet's veterinarian if your cat develops an injection-site lump that doesn't go away.
- **Decrease your pet's exposure to toxins.** Many older insecticides are not very safe. Some over-the-counter flea collars, for example, can increase cancer risk. Use newer, safer flea products prescribed by your veterinarian. In general, it is a good idea to reduce your use of lawn chemicals, fire-retardant chemicals in fabrics, and other chemically laden products in and around your home. Using "green" or natural products in your home, such as low-VOC paint and formaldehyde-free building materials, protects animals as well as humans. Read labels carefully—even "natural" products such as limonella, essential oils, and potpourri are toxic to cats.

DENTISTRY

In my opinion, dental care has saved the lives of more pets than almost any other advance in the field of veterinary medicine in the past 50 years. Promoting dental care to your clients is one of the most crucial things you will do as a veterinary team member. It has been shown that 80 percent of dogs and 70 percent of cats over the age of three have some degree of periodontal disease (Wiggs and Loprise 1997). Smaller dogs and cats live 15 to 20 percent longer if they receive dental care as needed throughout their lives. Larger dogs live 10 to 15 percent longer (Loesche 1994; DeBowes et al. 1996; Debowes 1992).

Tooth resorption is another very common problem. It is seen in 30 to 70 percent of cats and a smaller percentage of dogs (Van Wessum et al. 1992). These painful root and crown lesions eat away at a pet's teeth and require radiographs and extraction to treat.

> **Be an advocate for the pet.**

Dentistry provides profitable income for your practice, and it's one of the most common and important ways in which we can relieve pain and suffering in pets.

Sometimes it is difficult to show the owner dental problems in a pet's mouth. Cats' mouths are very small, dogs are often wiggly, lips get in the way, and the owner doesn't clearly understand what to look for. Teaching about dental care is a great opportunity to use pictures, exam-room PowerPoint presentations, DVDs, and models. Invest in a little pointer to pick out targeted lesions on the model or picture—it looks more polished and professional than using a pen. Keep some dental instruments in the exam-room drawers to demonstrate what will be done or how problems are diagnosed. Many people enjoy learning about their pets' health if the explanation is interesting and understandable. This is especially appropriate if there are school-age children in the room. They usually love learning about animals and nature, and they could become important members of their pets' health-care team.

> Remember, different people learn best in different ways.

One of the least expensive but most effective ways you can wow your clients is to take before-and-after pictures when you clean their pets' teeth. Capture images of any lesions that you find as well. These images can become part of

---

WHAT IS PERIODONTAL DISEASE?

Periodontal disease is characterized by progressive loss or destruction of the tissues around the teeth—the gingiva (i.e., gums)—the ligaments that hold the teeth in the bones, and the bones themselves. The usual progression is from gingivitis, where just the gums are infected, to the periodontal ligaments and bone. Gingivitis is reversible, but periodontitis (inflammation of the ligaments and bone) is not. Once the bone has receded and the teeth are loose there is no going back. The ligaments will never regrow, and once a tooth is loose it must be extracted in order for the bone and gums to heal.

Periodontal disease is not only the most common disease in dogs and cats but also one of the most preventable. Prevention consists of "dental nutrition," which includes a pet's basic diet as well as treats and appropriate chews; dental home care, which includes brushing the teeth and using plaque barriers, mouth rinses, and special chew toys; and dental cleaning, which means dental scaling and polishing under anesthesia when tartar buildup warrants it. This three-pronged approach can greatly reduce plaque and tartar buildup, which in turn reduces the risk of periodontal disease.

the patient's computerized medical record, so they also provide documentation of what was done and why. Dental care can get expensive, but having pictures to show how much was accomplished helps clients feel they got their money's worth. Make sure clients get to see their pets' dental radiographs. Customers always feel better about the money they've spent if they can see what it was they paid for.

In the exam room, don't be wishy-washy when talking about the dental care your patients require: Use the word "need": "Ms. Smith, the doctor says that Buffy needs a dental cleaning if she is to stay healthy for the next few years. When would you like to schedule that?" Do not say you recommend it or suggest it. These terms are too soft and imply that the procedure might not really be necessary.

Many clients have fears about anesthesia for their pets when dental care is done. With modern anesthetics and the availability of pre-anesthetic blood screening and sophisticated intraoperative monitors, these fears usually are unfounded. Assure your clients that the risk of untreated dental disease, especially periodontal disease, is far greater than the risk from anesthesia, and carefully explain the safety procedures and monitoring that will be done for the pet. You can assure Ms. Smith that Buffy will live a much healthier life because she is having the dental procedure done.

Sometimes you will call clients to schedule a dental cleaning. If they defer the procedure because of its cost, be sure to offer whatever financial options your clinic provides. Also make sure they are not actually declining because they have other fears or concerns. Many times the cost is used as a smokescreen to hide the fact that the client really doesn't have a good understanding of why dental care is needed or what is being accomplished for the amount you are quoting. You can use a phrase such as "Is the price the only thing that is stopping you from scheduling the procedure?"

If the client still hedges, say something like, "We don't want Buffy to be in pain from infected gums and teeth. Her life expectancy could be shortened. When do you think you would be able to schedule this needed care and we will call you back at that time?" Then be sure you do.

Occasionally, the owner will adamantly refuse care. The solution in these cases is to attempt to get the owner to do some home care, in the hopes that it will soon become obvious that it doesn't work and the client will return for the care the pet needed in the first place. Let's use Buffy again. If Ms. Smith doesn't think she wants to have Buffy's teeth cleaned, ask her if she would be able to brush Buffy's teeth, use a chlorhexidine mouth rinse, or rub her teeth daily with a washcloth. These procedures get the owner looking into and smelling the pet's mouth. The more the owner looks in the mouth, the more conscious she will be of the disease there. If there is redness, explain that red means pain: "If the gum is red, it is infected and painful." You can also schedule a no-charge follow-up oral exam visit a few weeks later to readdress the subject. It should be clear by then that what the owner has tried at home was not successful, and you may be able to then schedule the cleaning.

> *Red means pain: If the gum is red, it is infected and painful.*

This is not to say that home dental care is not effective. Veterinary team members should not only be extolling the virtues of tooth brushing to their clients, they should be teaching them how to brush their pets' teeth. Teach owners to start handling their puppies' or kittens' mouths during their very first visit to your hospital. At a subsequent visit, teach them how to brush the teeth effectively and what products to use. Mention dental care every time the owner comes in for a routine visit, remembering that clients need lots of repetition to buy into a service or product.

The Veterinary Oral Health Council examines evidence for the effectiveness of oral health products and grants its seal of approval when there is proof that a product actually works. Teach clients to look for the VOHC seal of approval. (See www.vohc.org/accepted_products.htm.)

> *The Veterinary Oral Health Council examines evidence for the effectiveness of oral health products. . . . Teach clients to look for the VOHC seal of approval.*

Discuss tartar-control diets, the importance of tartar-control treats, the number of treats the owner can feed the pet per day without lowering the pet's overall nutrition, and what chew toys are helpful. All these things are good preventive measures. All the brushing in the world won't cure a resorptive lesion or periodontal disease when it is present, however. Even with regular brushing, pets, just like people, still need regular dental cleanings to keep a healthy mouth.

Good scientific evidence exists for the use of a few specific dental home care products. These include therapeutic dental diets, tooth brushing, chlorhexidine for dogs (available as mouth rinses and gels, impregnated rawhide chews, and toothpastes) and zinc ascorbate rinses in cats, and certain dental treats. Evidence for many other products is scant or lacking altogether. When in doubt, look for the VOHC logo or seal on the product packaging or ask the veterinarians in your clinic what they recommend. The VOHC is administered by the American Veterinary Dental College and reviews the results of tests on dental products performed in accordance with approved protocols. If you see that seal, there is at least some sort of scientific evidence that supports the use of that product.

You will always have those clients who simply decline everything you offer them, from tooth brushing to extractions. In these cases, the best you can do is to make sure they understand the consequences. The consequences are usually not as bad for large-breed dogs as for small dogs, unless a tooth is broken or abscessed. In small breeds that are prone to periodontal disease, lack of dental care has severe health risks for the affected pet. Cats are all over the board. We see 15-year-old cats with great teeth and three-year-olds with advanced periodontal disease. The more disease is present, the more likely it is that lack of dental care will shorten a pet's life expectancy.

If Buffy already has a mouthful of infected teeth, you do need to come right out and tell the owner that this is a painful disease. How can the client make good, informed decisions if he or she does not realize the scope of the pet's problem? Withholding treatment for a painful illness of any kind, whether it is an unrepaired broken leg, severe and chronic ear infections, or cancer, is not fair to the animal. It is the job of health-care professionals to tell the owners the truth about their pets, even when it is bad news. Many, many people think that as long as a dog is not whimpering, it is not in pain. But animals often suffer silently. It is your job to speak for the animal and tell the owner when the pet hurts.

Generally, the doctor is the one delivering this sort of awkward information. But you can and should back up what the doctor has said with the way that you suggest follow-up appointments or provide further information about the problem and its treatment. Try: "Ms. Smith, this is painful for your pet and greatly affects her quality of life, just as it would yours." There's nothing that sours the day more than watching a pet owner walk out the door when you know he or she will never comply with the veterinarian's recommendations and the pet will continue to suffer. This situation is exactly what we want to prevent. We should try hard to teach clients about caring for their pet properly before it's time to deliver bad news.

To help your client empathize with the pet, you can relate the pet's health to human health. Studies have been shown that pregnant women with periodontal disease are seven times more likely to have a premature or low-birth-weight baby, and that people with periodontal disease are twice as likely to have heart attacks. Just like in humans, periodental disease in pets can lead to serious health problems.

If the client agrees to your dental-care health plan, explain carefully what will be done during the procedure. Many clients don't realize that it involves anesthesia, or that you perform an ultrasonic scaling, polish, and fluoride or sealer treatment, and often full-mouth X-rays, just as their own dentists do for them. Detail what is being done and what your clinic's policy is in case a problem, such as a fractured tooth, is discovered during the procedure. At the end of this section you will find a form that you can use on the morning that the patient is admitted for the dental procedure. It requires a client signature. Sometimes it helps to remind pet owners that dental care performed early and often is cheaper than dental care performed later. If payment plans are available, be sure that your clients know this.

Notice the check-off lines on the form giving the owner a choice in how the doctor should proceed if a problem is found. Sometimes, even when the owner is waiting for your call, you cannot get through because the owner is on another phone call or stepped out for the mail. Make sure you know the correct phone number to call and whose number it is.

You may become frustrated when dealing with a client who does not fully understand what it is that needs to be done during a procedure and then is shocked at the final bill or upset that you didn't explain better. The way to prevent this situation is to make sure the client has heard you when you present information. Even if you tell the client in the exam room that Buffy may need to have a few teeth removed because of periodontal disease or resorptive lesions, the client may not fully grasp that information. The client may be busy thinking about a pet who died under anesthesia 20 years ago. Be sure you have gone over the form with the owner in detail before he or she signs it. A client cannot be considered to have given informed consent for any procedure until he or she has actually been informed!

> **Be honest with your clients and don't surprise them.**

Many times we assume clients understand far more about medical procedures than they really do. Half of our clients are medically illiterate—they may have very little understanding of medical terminology or how the body functions. Most don't know what a periodontal ligament is. We need to teach them what our treatment plan is, in simple terms.

We tend to use softer words sometimes so as not to frighten clients, such as "sedate" instead of "general anesthesia." The problem comes when Buffy dies under anesthesia or has complications the client wasn't warned about. When the doctor ends up in court because the owner sued and the client says, "They told me they were merely sedating her, not that she would be under general anesthesia for over an hour," the doctor will lose that battle. Explain clearly and in simple language what is involved in the procedure, what the risks and benefits are, and what will happen if an unexpected problem is encountered.

Dental procedures can be difficult to estimate because so many problems can't be seen when the pet is awake. Costs also vary depending on the size of the pet—a 10-day course of pain medication and antibiotics for an infected tooth can be costly, especially for a large dog. Give the client an estimate for any extra procedures, such as extractions, early on whenever possible. In many cases, you'll need to call the client to explain what needs to be done once the pet is anesthetized. If you've already informed him or her that extraction time, anesthesia, dental instrument pack, X-rays, and medications will cost X amount, the client will be better prepared for bad news and more likely to give consent. Always estimate high—clients will be far happier to pay less than the quote than to pay more. Don't forget to add the cost of pre-anesthetic blood work, electrocardiogram, or IV fluids to the estimate, as well as any home-care items you want to send home afterward.

Grading the teeth is an important part of a routine physical exam, because dental health is vital to overall health. For the medical files, it's best to record tartar, gingivitis, and other problems separately. This should be done each time a pet comes in for a routine exam. Both before and after the dental cleaning, always be sure that recheck exams are scheduled and that callbacks and reminders for future dental services are entered into the computer.

Before the patient goes home after a dental procedure, be sure a team member spends some time discussing follow-up care. Now that the pet's teeth are clean, it is the perfect time to start a regular routine of brushing. A change in diet and chew toys may also be appropriate. Most cats, and many dogs, will sound hoarse or congested for a few days after a dental procedure. Tell the owners what to expect when the pet arrives back home. Also, be sure to praise the client for having the procedure done—too many owners never do and their pets will suffer because of it.

The form included at the end of this section is one you can use for dental admissions. On the back of the form is another paragraph for the owner to initial that contains basic verbiage for any anesthesia consent form. This form uses language from *Legal Consents for Veterinary Practices*, Fourth Edition, by James F. Wilson (Priority Press, 2006). Be sure that anything you have a client sign has up-to-date legal language. Consent forms have two purposes—not only do they ensure the client is informed as to exactly what will be done, but they also protect the veterinary practice from liability.

RESOURCES

AAHA Dental Care Guidelines. www.healthypet.com/PetCare/PetCareArticle.aspx?art_key=53d99aad-e759-473e-8977-f8f75eefb754.

American Veterinary Dental College, www.AVDC.org.

American Veterinary Dental Society, www.avds-online.org.

Animal Dentistry and Oral Surgery Specialists, www.mypetsdentist.com/site/view/104382_PreparingmyPetfortheVisit.pml.

Boss, Nan. 2009. *How We Do Things Here*. Lakewood, CO: AAHA Press.

Butler-Schein Animal Health, www.accessbutler.com/logonu.asp. This company sells digital cameras, dental models, dental charts, dental chart pads, and lots of dental equipment.

DVM360, www.dvm360.com. This website has lots of dental materials. Under the "Business Center" menu, choose "Client Handouts" to find "Bad Breath (Halitosis) in Pets," "Dandy's Day at the Dentist," "Dental Disease Handout," "Slideshow: Show Clients How to Clean Pets' Teeth," "Guidelines for Dental Home Care," a form called "How Does Your Pet's Mouth Look" to fill out with clients, "How to Brush Your Pet's Teeth," "Caring for Your Pet's Teeth and Gums," and a dental admitting form. Under "Patient Care" you'll find "Do Not Neglect Dental Care: Talk to Clients About Brushing Their Pets' Teeth."

Hill's Pet Nutrition, Pet Dental Home, www.petdental.com/pd2/index.jsp?FOLDER%3C%3Efolder_id=1408474395185675&bmUID=1288468156375.

Shipp's Dental and Specialty Products, www.drshipp.com/. Shipp's sells many different dental models.

Smiles. A book of enlarged, color, before-and-after dental pictures, available from Pfizer (ask for Pfizer representative to obtain a copy).

Wilson, James F. 2006. *Legal Consents for Veterinary Practices*, 4th ed. Indianapolis: Priority Press.

"Worth a Thousand Words." 2007. *Veterinary Economics*, February 1.

HOSPITAL ADMISSION STATEMENT/AUTHORIZATION FOR TREATMENT

OWNER .... PET'S NAME .... DATE ....

Surgery/Procedure to be performed: Dental cleaning including IV fluids? ECG screening? Other Surgery needed?

Full-mouth X-rays?   Extractions: Possible but unlikely?   Likely?   Known to be needed? Other services needed while in hospital?

Nail Trim? HW Test? Fecal? UA? Vaccines? .... Microchip? ....

Other:

I understand that the dental care my pet will receive today includes general anesthesia. The teeth will be cleaned with an ultrasonic scaler, then polished and treated with chlorhexidine rinse and sealant. Each tooth will be probed and checked for cavities, gum recession or lesions, fractures, and periodontal disease. The nature of the procedure has been explained to me and no guarantee has been made as to the results or cure. I understand that there may be risk involved in these procedures.

Factors that limit our ability to detect every dental problem your pet may have ahead of time include:

1. Lack of patient cooperation to allow proper visualization, especially of the back teeth.
2. Many periodontal problems can be detected only by probing under the gum with an instrument.
3. Dental tartar can hide underlying cavities or fractures.
4. Some problems can be detected only with X-rays.

If further problems are detected while your pet is under anesthesia, how should they be handled? (Choose one of the following.)

☐ Perform whatever procedures are needed.

☐ Please call me.
  I will be available at the following telephone number(s): ....

If for some reason I am unavailable when you call, please:

☐ Perform whatever procedures are needed, or

☐ Do only what I have authorized. I understand my pet may have to undergo another anesthetic episode to complete the dental treatment.

ALL SERVICES OF THIS HOSPITAL ARE DONE ON A CASH BASIS AND MUST BE PAID BEFORE THE PET CAN BE RELEASED.

Estimated Total $ ....

Payment will be made by:

☐ Cash   ☐ Check   ☐ Visa   ☐ MasterCard   ☐ Discover   ☐ CareCredit

I have read and understand the above conditions of this hospital.

....
SIGNATURE OF OWNER OR RESPONSIBLE AGENT   **DATE**

Whom should we call in the event of problems?

NAME .... **PHONE** ....

Following the procedure, would you like to be updated with a text message or a phone call? ....

EMERGENCIES

When someone calls the clinic with an emergency, get enough information from the caller for the doctor and technician to be able to effectively assist when the patient arrives. You must ask for the client's complete name as well as the pet's name so that the patient's chart can be pulled. If the pet has medical problems, such as medication allergies, the doctor needs to know this to treat the animal properly when it arrives.

If the client has not been to the clinic before, get the species, breed, and approximate weight of the pet. Ask how long it will take for the client to drive to the clinic, what condition the pet is in, and if the owner knows where the clinic is located.

Do not ask the client what happened. If the pet needs immediate care, letting the client launch into a long story about how the injury occurred is not helpful. You need to stay calm and businesslike while still keeping your voice tone empathetic. Get the information you need the most, and get it quickly, so that the pet will be able to get the care it needs as soon as possible.

Sometimes the client believes there is an emergency but the situation does not sound critical to the veterinary team member who has answered the telephone. When this happens, treat the situation as an emergency anyway. Do not try to diagnose over the telephone—perhaps in the stress of the moment, the client is not giving you all the information. It is not appropriate to tell the client that he or she is overreacting.

THE EMERGENCY VISIT

When the patient arrives, the doctor and the technician or assistant need to focus on that patient. The receptionist or another team member needs to focus on the client.

Keep in mind that there is a big difference between the client's perspective and that of the veterinary team. You've probably seen worse, but the client probably hasn't. You need to be reassuring and let the client know you are taking him or her seriously, even if it doesn't seem like the injury or problem is severe. A torn toenail can bleed profusely. To the client, it is an emergency.

> **Look and act professional.**

Move the client and patient into an exam room as soon as possible. If the pet is hurt badly and taken to the treatment area, the owner may become more upset watching the necessary procedures being done. Your script goes something like: "This isn't an easy thing to see. Some of our procedures to help Fluffy won't look pleasant. We're happy to keep you informed if you'd like to wait here."

If the client insists on being present and the medical team decides to comply, the doctor may need to make it clear that the client must do exactly as told and stay calm. Otherwise, the client may hinder the work and the team may not be able to help the patient as much as possible.

> **Remember the Golden Rule.**

Be understanding and reassuring while the doctors and techs are working on the patient. Remember the tips in the introduction about empathizing with clients. Tell the client that the team is doing the best they can and the pet is in good hands. Never say anything that implies that the pet owner or the person who brought in the pet is at fault for the illness or injury. The person feels bad enough already.

When the doctor has had a chance to assess the pet's injuries, the owner may need to make some decisions about the pet's care. However, many owners at this point are not thinking clearly. To get them to focus better, use a script like this: "This must be terrible for you. I can understand how distressing it is to see your pet be hit by a car. We're going to do everything we can *and* we need you to make some decisions." Use "and" here (not "but") to avoid sounding patronizing.

Emergency care can be very costly. Clients frequently accuse veterinary team members of being heartless for discussing monetary issues in an emergency situation. Because the costs can easily mount into the hundreds of dollars within minutes, however, this discussion is a necessity. Tell the client: "I know this seems harsh, but we need to know how much care you can authorize us to perform. Buffy's charges may run over $500 and we need to know if it is okay to proceed. Our manager is here to discuss the financial aspects if you wish."

You may need to fill out an authorization form quickly for the client to sign. Be realistic and professional when discussing the costs of needed care. When the dust settles, the clinic accounts receivable manager is going to be very unhappy if the bill goes unpaid. Don't let yourself get caught up in the client's anguish and forget that paying for care is part of owning a pet.

> **Don't get defensive.**

If at all possible, have a team member stay with the distraught client at all times. Ask if a friend or family member could be called for support, and give the owner frequent updates to avoid frantic or overly assertive behavior. Remember that time drags for clients who are agitated and full of adrenaline. If the prognosis for the patient looks poor, be sure the client is told as soon as possible. Refer to the "Grief Counseling and Euthanasia" section in this book for more information on communicating with clients who have lost a pet.

Ideally, the patient lives, the client pays the bill, and everyone lives happily ever after. If the pet dies, however, the owner may need the undivided attention of a team member. One of the kindest things we do for clients is supporting them through the grief of losing a pet. Clients are often very appreciative later on for the time and effort you have spent to help them through a tough time.

Consider having first aid seminars for your clients, using videotapes and demonstrating on stuffed animals. Or call your local emergency clinic for handouts or suggestions on handling emergency care and transport. They may also have a clinician or technician on staff who can present a seminar on emergency protocols for veterinary team members or clients.

Be sure you also have phone numbers available for your local poison control hotline so you can refer clients there who call you with questions about poisoning. Often pet owners call because they are worried that a pet has eaten something dangerous, and your entire team should be prepared to handle these situations.

THE EMERGENCY REFERRAL

Years ago, veterinary clinics saw most of their own emergencies because emergency pet hospitals were rare. Now there is pretty good access to emergency and specialty care for most urban and suburban practices, and even for many rural ones. Specialty medicine has grown by orders of magnitude, so we have had to learn how to refer clients to specialists as well as how to explain to them why we are referring them.

There is still some resistance to referring on the part of some veterinarians, who have fears that clients who are referred will see their primary veterinarian as less than competent. Doctors may worry that the referral hospital won't deliver customer service as good as theirs, or that the specialist will say something derogatory about them. Additionally, the veterinarians at a general practice may not trust the doctors at a nearby specialty hospital.

It's the responsibility of both the referring doctors and the referral doctors to communicate effectively in order to deliver the best possible care to their mutual clients and patients. As you assist with referrals, you will likely have conversations with the team members of the referral practice that are similar to the ones you have with clients whose pets have a serious problem, only in reverse. You will be telling the referral practice team about the pet being referred, sending over medical records, and the like. In an emergency situation this may mean faxing records or communicating essential details over the telephone.

There are three types of referring doctors: (1) those who want to send the pet to the specialist and have the specialist take over all care decisions; (2) those who want to send patients for specific services, such as CT, but want to maintain all control over the case as a whole; and (3) those who want to communicate and collaborate with the specialist. Be honest with the team at the referral practice and tell them what your doctor wants or expects from them. This will make the relationship go more smoothly.

You will also need to explain the reason for the referral to the client. Most clients understand that there are things outside the realm of expertise of the general practitioner. Explain carefully what the doctor's expectations are for the care of the pet by that facility, give the client an idea of how much it will cost, and express your trust in the referral doctors. All of this may need to be done very quickly in an emergency situation. Explain the need for the referral calmly and with a confident tone. The client will only feel comfortable with the new specialist doctor if you are.

It's also important to explain how your practice, the specialist, and the client will be communicating during the time the pet is in the specialist's care. Be sure the referral doctors know that they can call your clinic anytime if they need more information or want to confer with the veterinarian on a case, and that your clinic expects a phone call following the surgery or procedure for an update on how things are going. If the client already knows you and other members of your team, he or she may feel more comfortable calling you with questions or for help in making decisions than discussing it with the new veterinarian. If you have the latest information on the pet's condition, you will be better equipped to help. Make sure that these follow-up reports are added to the patient's chart.

The client may also call you because he or she does not understand the treatment or options the referral hospital has recommended or performed. Sometimes this is because the referral hospital team didn't do a good job communicating with the client, but many times it's just because the client was overwhelmed, or not always thinking clearly. Clients often believe your veterinarians will have a better perspective on the situation because they know them and their pets better than the referral doctor does.

Clients may also worry about making the wrong decision in an emergency situation. Often decisions about treatment need to be made quickly, without time to think things through as carefully as the pet owner might like. Whatever it is they decide to do, and whoever ends up talking to them, clients should always be positively reinforced for their choices. In other words, even if you would or wouldn't euthanize or treat your own pet the same way in the same circumstances, you must always try to tell the client that you understand why he or she made a particular choice and that it's the best thing for their family and pet. You could say, "I think this is a good choice for you and for Fluffy . . ." or "I think you'll feel better knowing that you did all you could . . ." Treat people like responsible, caring adults who will make responsible, caring choices, and that's usually what they will do.

RESOURCES

DVM360, www.dvm360.com. DVM360 has a referral form you can use. Look in "Patient Care Forms" under the "Business Center" menu.

Lagoni, Laurel, and Dana Durrance. 2010. *Connecting with Clients: Practical Communication Techniques for 15 Common Situations*, 2nd ed. Lakewood, CO: AAHA Press.

FLEAS AND TICKS AND OTHER THINGS THAT BITE

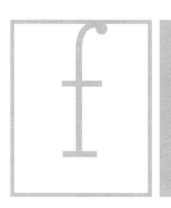

The "cat flea," *Ctenocephalides felis*, is the most common external parasite of dogs and cats in North America. Most clients know very little about them, however. This creates confusion and disappointment on the part of clients when fleas become a problem. Once clients have to deal with fleas, and find out they could easily have been prevented, they may wish the veterinary team had said something about them beforehand. The team must work together to communicate a consistent, coherent message about flea prevention and control.

Infestation with fleas can result in a number of problems for pets, including itching, hair loss, anemia, and tapeworms. That's why it's so much better to prevent fleas than to wait until an infestation occurs. Often, however, clients don't want to hear about flea control until they already have fleas on the pet or in their home. This avoidance attitude can make our job challenging. But if we look at flea education as an opportunity to make learning fun, it is possible to break through these barriers.

When fleas bite pets, they cause an itchy allergic reaction that can become quite severe. Fleas carry viral and bacterial diseases and *Mycoplasma haemofelis* (formerly known as *Haemobartonella*), a blood parasite in cats. Moreover, in small animals, especially puppies and kittens, the anemia that fleas cause from feeding on the animal's blood can be fatal. Fleas also carry tapeworms, which, when ingested by the pet during grooming, will mature and multiply in the pet's digestive tract. Teach your clients to watch for these parasites (see the "Intestinal Parasites" section).

Fleas actually can be rather fascinating. People love to learn about nature and science when the subject is presented in an interesting way. Show enthusiasm for the amazing facts about fleas, and your clients will be more attentive. It's fun to show children and adults pictures or models of fleas and their life cycle, "ooh and ahh" over their ugliness, and come up with a diabolical plan to get rid of them.

FASCINATING FACTS ABOUT FLEAS

There are over 2,000 flea species in the world. Fleas can perform the human equivalent of jumping over St. Paul's Cathedral in London . . . not just once but 600 times an hour for three days in a row! Here are some other amazing facts you can share with your clients:

- Fleas have a ball of a substance called resilin above their hind legs. This is what gives them their bounce. Resilin is the most elastic substance known. A resilin ball dropped from 100 feet would bounce back to 97 feet!
- One theory says that lap dogs were bred not for their company but to distract fleas—it was hoped that fleas would bite the dogs instead of their owners. Modern life makes it easy to forget about fleas. Our houses are drier than those of our ancestors, and flea larvae need moisture to reproduce. Hence we are less plagued with them than our forebears. However, for most of history humans of all classes were routinely flea-bitten.
- Bat fleas in Southeast Asia hitch rides to the bat roosts on the backs of bat earwigs. As many as 41 fleas have been counted on the back of one earwig.
- An Antarctic flea has evolved to wait nine months under several feet of ice and snow for its host, the petrel, to return to the nest.
- London's Natural History Museum contains a collection of souvenirs from nineteenth-century Mexico of "dressed fleas"—tiny, meticulously dressed figures of a woodcutter, a drummer boy, a wedding couple, and the like. Made of tiny bits of cloth and paper, they have flea heads for faces.

Use some imagination and creativity and think of ways to entertain and educate clients about parasites. Set up a display in your waiting room, hang flea cutouts from the ceiling, or give a talk at your local humane society on fleas, ticks, and other parasites. Explain the new flea products that are available during your talks. Technology has come a long way since the old dips and powders, and this is a fine opportunity to brag about the great products your hospital has for flea control and how simple and safe they are for both the client and the pet. By and large, the products sold by veterinarians are safer and more effective than most available over-the-counter treatments.

Chemicals such as permethrin and pyrethrin, the main ingredients in older flea and tick preventive products, were developed in the 1970s. They are neurotoxins that affect mammals as well as insects, so they can be toxic to pets, especially cats. In addition, since they've been around for 40 years or more, fleas and ticks have become resistant to them. The patents for these chemicals have long since expired, so they are inexpensive and readily available, but they are much more risky for both humans and animals and they often are ineffective. Newer products are more expensive but they work much better and are far less toxic than permethrins.

The Environmental Protection Agency received 44,000 reports of adverse reactions to over-the-counter permethrin and pyrethrin flea products in 2008, including 600 deaths. Side effects from these products included vomiting, diarrhea, tremors, seizures, eye redness, coughing, and other problems. Often people do not read or follow the instructions on the label. Many of these reactions were the result of cats being exposed to dog products, or people using products on pets that were smaller or younger than those for which the product was intended. These adverse-reaction statistics explain why it's so important for us to help pet owners choose the most effective and safest products, and to carefully explain how to use them properly.

Consumers tend to think that if a product is available at the grocery store, it's safe, but this is not always true. New flea products generally are released for prescription use first and eventually go over-the-counter as their patents run out. Each generation of products is safer, more effective, and easier to use than the previous one—and some of the newer over-the-counter products are fine—but clients cannot tell which products are safe and effective and which are not. The flea-control products that veterinarians provide are generally the most effective and safest available. Another factor is that black-market and counterfeit goods have infiltrated the OTC market, whereas veterinarians buy products directly from the manufacturer, eliminating that possibility. In 2009 the EPA began a yearlong safety review of flea products, subsequently recommending stronger label warnings, public education, and increased monitoring.

TOP 10 MISTAKES PET OWNERS MAKE WHEN TRYING TO CONTROL FLEAS (THAT WE CAN TEACH THEM NOT TO MAKE)

1. Waiting until they actually see fleas on the dog or cat before beginning treatment. By the time you see fleas on a pet, the fleas have had ample time to reproduce. There are thousands of eggs and pupae—all potential new fleas.
2. Treating just the dog, just the cat, or only outdoor dogs and cats. All of the dogs and cats in the household must be treated.
3. Not using flea products at the prescribed intervals. To maintain effectiveness, the product must be used at specified intervals. Be sure that your client understands your instructions and decides on a method of remembering when to repeat the application (such as a note on his or her calendar or BlackBerry).
4. Blaming a cat's or dog's fleas on birds, rabbits, or squirrels, or on the boarding kennel or veterinary clinic. Fleas don't jump from one animal to another; they jump from the nest area directly onto the pet. Once they have found a host animal they stay on that animal. If a cat or dog has fleas, the pet has come into contact with an area in which fleas were hatching. It did not get the fleas in the hospital or from the pet in the cage next door.
5. Believing that any old store-bought flea collar will keep fleas away. Some over-the-counter products contain chemicals that are less safe and less effective than products sold by veterinarians.
6. Incorrectly applying topical flea-control products. Show the client how to apply the product.
7. Thinking dogs and cats do not need flea control if they are outside only in an enclosed area or are wearing a leash or harness. Fences and harnesses do not provide flea protection.

8. Using flea-control products only in the summer. Products need to be used consistently during the entire flea season—which in warmer parts of the country is all year round.
9. Having unrealistic expectations of flea-control products. Fleas take hours to die from topical flea-control products, not seconds or minutes. As fleas hatch out and jump on the pet, they will slowly die, but you may still see live fleas even on treated pets. This doesn't mean the product isn't working. Growth-preventive medications like Sentinel do not in fact cause adult fleas to die at all; they prevent eggs from hatching. We need to carefully explain how these products work to avoid disappointment on the part of the pet owner.
10. Not identifying and removing flea hiding places in the home and yard. Clients need to be taught how to rid their home and yard of flea nest sites.

It is easier to prevent fleas than to treat them. Using flea-control measures on the pet is safer for the family—and especially for any babies or toddlers in the house—than treating the whole house with insecticides. With the flea products available now, there is no reason clients should have to go through the hassle of a full-blown flea infestation. Sell them on a preventive program, and they will be grateful never to have to go through that. With all of the great flea products available now, we have a wealth of resources for clients, and they are an important source of income for a practice.

It is a good idea to have a client handout detailing the prevention and treatment products available at your clinic and their prices. Be familiar with these items and their benefits and drawbacks, as well as their costs, so you can offer the best solutions for each pet. You also need to know exactly what to recommend for major flea infestations. Fogging or exterminating a home can be costly, and if it is not done properly, clients will need to repeat the process. If you gave them improper advice, they will probably take their business elsewhere.

Modern-day flea products control fleas by breaking the flea life cycle in one or more places. This is essentially an attempt to force fleas to extinction in a localized environment such as the house or yard. If the intervals between treatments are too long (in other words, the client forgets to apply the topical flea preventive on the first of the month and instead remembers it two weeks later), or a treatment is completely missed, the fleas can survive long enough to reproduce and start their life cycle again. On again, off again treatment programs rarely work, regardless of the product used. Treatment failures are usually due to improper use or application or unrealistic expectations on the part of the pet owner.

Most of your clients don't know the flea's life cycle, what flea dirt looks like, or even what a flea or tick looks like. It is common for clients to bring pets in for examination of a lump that is actually a tick, or even to ask to have a tick removed that is actually a lump. This is one of those occasions when it is easy to sound flippant or dismissive. (You may say, "Oh, that's a tick," but the tone of voice says, "Boy, are you stupid. Anyone can see that's a tick!") Don't let yourself slip. This may be old hat to you, but for the client this is all new. Now is the time to wow them with your helpfulness and teaching skills, not to sound bored, expressionless, or patronizing.

Always be diplomatic when discussing fleas. Many clients think fleas are only a problem if their house is dirty, and they are deeply embarrassed to have a flea problem at all. "My dog has never had fleas!" You must reassure them that fleas are not a bad reflection on them. One hundred years ago or more, before everyone had central heating and air conditioning (which keep the air drier and thus reduce the survival of flea larvae), vacuum cleaners (which suck up flea eggs), and insecticides, everyone had fleas. In many parts of the world, they still do. In the United States, we are lucky enough to be able to keep fleas outdoors, for the most part. Sooner or later, however, anyone can wind up with them, even households without pets. Wildlife and stray animals bring fleas into the yard, and fleas can hop long distances looking for a meal. They are small enough to come in through window screens, and they are happy to hitch a ride in on people's shoes and clothing.

Despite many effective flea-control products on the market today, many owners still struggle with flea infestations on their dogs and cats. A flea infestation is more than just a few fleas on the pet. With an infestation, adult fleas on the pet are actively reproducing, and all of the flea life stages (eggs, larvae, pupae, and adults) are present in areas the pet frequents. The source of infestation may not be the client's own pet. It could be a neighbor's dog, a stray cat or raccoon nesting in a garage or shed, the dog park, or anywhere the dog or cat goes. Adult fleas jump onto pets as they pass by. These hitchhiker fleas then have the potential to reproduce and create a new infestation in the home or yard. An adult female flea can lay hundreds of eggs within a few days. Using preventives properly ensures that the fleas will die before they get that chance.

Clients who live in certain geographical areas may be surprised to learn that some kinds of insects are a concern in their area. You may need to explain that many insect and arachnid species are expanding their ranges. This is due to climate change, habitat modification by humans, and our mobile lifestyles. Ticks are now a big problem in parts of the country that, formerly didn't see them very often. Heartworm disease slowly spread north from its origins in the southeastern United States and is now found in every one of the 50 states. Other insect-borne diseases are also spreading today.

> **Think of yourself as a teacher.**

Ticks carry several serious diseases, including Lyme disease, ehrlichiosis, Rocky Mountain spotted fever, and anaplasmosis. In a recent survey done by Idexx Laboratories, half of all U.S. states reported more than 500 Lyme-positive dogs, according to the Centers for Disease Control and Prevention. April is "Prevent Lyme Disease" month, and that makes it a good time to make a special effort to educate people in your community about ticks.

Not only do we need to educate clients about the parasites themselves, we need to explain what those other diseases are that are often included in heartworm tests, and we need to have a protocol in place for positives. Have handouts for clients to explain the diseases you are testing for and what should be done in case of a positive test. You will likely be the one to talk with the client when the test results come in to explain what the results mean. If a test is positive, you will need to give the client an appropriate handout and get the client's okay to do a complete blood count (CBC). A CBC is needed to test for thrombocytopenia, or low platelet count, when a pet tests positive for *Anaplasma* on an in-house test. The doctor will likely get involved only if the pet is sick—if the CBC comes back the next day showing thrombocytopenia, the doctor will want to call the owner to discuss the results and the treatment. In a healthy dog with a normal CBC, however, the veterinarian may not need to speak with the client at all. Instead, the veterinary assistants and technicians will handle much of the communication that is needed in this case.

> ### April is "Prevent Lyme Disease" month . . . and that makes it a good time to make a special effort to educate people in your community about ticks.

It's important to make sure the client knows how to use any product or medication before leaving your clinic with it. Research shows that resistance to insecticides isn't nearly as big a problem as clients making mistakes in choosing and applying flea and tick products (Dryden and Rust 1994). Clients may have trouble with even simple tasks, such as properly opening or perforating the tube of the product. They forget to reapply it, don't read the directions, or stop or start too early or late in the season. Injury and death to pets from improper pesticide application are all too common. You must also explain that a topical insecticide takes time to work and that the client may still see parasites on the pet while the process is under way.

You may need to explain vaccinations for tick-borne diseases as well, depending on what your clinic's protocols are. Although flea and tick prevention seems like a simple topic, it's not. Your clients need you to take the time this important topic deserves to discuss it with them, because it's an area in which mistakes and misconceptions abound.

A few other parasites are worth mentioning as well. You will sometimes get questions about head lice. Lice are very species-specific. In other words, cattle, horse, and dog lice each only parasitize that specific species. Dog lice don't like people and human lice don't like any of these animals. Children with head lice *did not* get them from the family pet.

Demodectic and Cheyletiella mites are also host-specific. Sarcoptic mites, however, are contagious to both people and pets. So is ringworm, a fungal infection. Fleas will bite people, especially children, as well as dogs and cats.

Because people can pick up skin problems from their pets, dogs and cats with itchy skin should be seen by a doctor for appropriate diagnosis and treatment. This is both a selling point for your hospital and good advice for the health of the family members who live with a pet. Be careful not to make it sound as if pets are dirty beasts that carry dreadful diseases on a daily basis—you don't want the client to have the pet euthanized because it might make the baby sick—but do explain that taking care of the pet promptly may also protect the family.

RESOURCES

Blagburn B. L., and M. W. Dryden. 2009. "Biology, Treatment and Control of Flea and Tick Infestations." *Veterinary Clinics of North America: Small Animal Practice* 39, no. 6 (November): 1173–1200.

Blagburn, B. L., M. W. Dryden, P. Payne, M. K. Rust, D. E. Jacobs, R. Bond, M. J. Huchinson, et al. 2006. "New Methods and Strategies for Monitoring Susceptibility of Fleas to Current Flea Control Products." *Veterinary Therapeutics* 7, no. 2 (Summer): 86–98.

Centers for Disease Control and Prevention. For information on the incidence of Lyme disease, see cdc.gov/ncidod/dvbod/Lyme/Id_Incidence.htm. For a Lyme disease risk map, see cdc.gov/ncidod/dvbod/Lyme/riskmap.htm.

Companion Animal Parasite Council, www.capcvet.org. This site has lots of good information, including parasite treatment and prevention protocols. The companion website at www.petsandparasites.org is for pet owners.

Dryden, M. W., and M. K. Rust. 1994. "The Cat Flea—Biology, Ecology and Control." *Veterinary Parasitology* 52, nos. 1–2 (March): 1–19.

Dvm360, Parasitology Center, http://veterinarycalendar.dvm360.com/avhc/Parasitology+Center/home/47731. Do a search from this page on "Canine and Feline Demodicosis" for up-to-date information on Demodex mites. Other articles and interactive quizzes can also be found on the site. Under the "Business Center" menu, choose "Patient Care Forms" to find "Don't Get Ticked at Ticks—Get Even," a chart of selected parasiticides for dogs and cats, and a "Flea Control History Form." Under "Client Handouts" you'll find "Lyme Disease and Your Dog," "Demodicosis in Dogs," "Ivermectin for the Treatment of Demodicosis," and "Top 10 Flea Myths."

Little, S. E., et al. 2010. "Lyme Borreliosis in Dogs and Humans in the USA." *Trends in Parasitology* 26, no. 4 (March): 213–218.

GRIEF COUNSELING AND EUTHANASIA

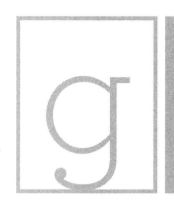

Eighty percent of pet owners consider their pets family members. Anyone who has loved a pet and lost it knows that the sadness that comes with saying goodbye can be very painful. It is not unusual for the grief following the death of a pet to be as intense as the grief following the death of a human loved one. For many children, it is their first experience with grief and loss. Losing a pet is a traumatic experience for most clients, and this emotional time deserves special attention. How you handle euthanasia and grieving clients says a lot about how much you care and leaves a lasting impression on the client.

The doctor needs to help the client make the decision whether to euthanize or not, but anyone on the team may need to explain the different options for cremation, describe how the euthanasia solution will be administered, or ask whether the owner wants a clay paw print. Sometimes the explanations are done over the phone by the client relations specialist (CRS); if not, these may be done in the exam room by an assistant or technician. There is no law that says a veterinarian needs to do the euthanasia—technicians are perfectly capable, and in humane societies anyone can get certified to perform euthanasia by taking a class. However, in most practices the doctors administer the euthanasia solution and do at least some of the counseling and comforting of the client.

We don't always know when a patient comes in that euthanasia is going to end up happening. Many times, though, we already know that a pet has a fatal disease. If the client calls about a pet we already know is terminal, the CRS who answers the phone and schedules the appointment may be the one who ends up talking to the clients about how they are feeling or whether the time is right. The CRS or assistant may be the one who calls the clients when the pet's ashes are ready to be picked up, or sees the clients when they come in to get them. These are also times when the clients may need emotional support.

Pay special attention to children at this time. Children are prone to certain misconceptions about the subject of death and are often keenly aware that something is not right with the pet. An honest approach is best when dealing with a child, who also needs to know that his or her feelings and opinions have been listened to before a pet is put down. Parents who try to hide death from their children should be counseled that children need time to say goodbye. This is also a wonderful opportunity to teach children about the permanence of death and the rituals involved in loss.

Children younger than five years old have difficulty understanding the finality of death. They may need several explanations, long after the pet is gone, as to why it does not come back. This age group also takes words literally, so it is best not to use the phrase "put to sleep" with young children.

From ages five to nine, children tend to perceive death as a punishment. They must be reassured that the pet did not die because of something the parents or the children themselves did or did not do.

After age nine, most children have a more realistic concept of death and can understand religious or philosophical ideas about it. Participating in a burial or memorial service for the pet, if possible, can make children feel better. Suggest this to your clients when it is appropriate to do so.

Adults should not try to hide their sorrow in front of their children. If adult clients let themselves show their grief, children know that feelings of sadness are normal. Talking about the pet after its death is also wise. The pet deserves to be remembered as a part of the family and one of the children's most wonderful friends.

Adults may need help coping as well. Society does not always provide the support people need after the traumatic loss of a pet, especially if the pet was an important source of comfort for its owner. When humans die, relatives and friends usually provide a great deal of support and sympathy, which helps the bereaved through the initial mourning period. Unfortunately, this support is often not forthcoming on the death of a pet. Veterinary team members can help by offering gestures such as sympathy cards or notes, sending flowers, or calling the client after the euthanasia to ask how things are going.

For the elderly, the loss of a pet may be particularly difficult. A pet may be an elderly person's only companion and a major source of meaning in his or her life. Adopting another pet may be impossible if the owner will soon need nursing care or is not able to train a young pet and help it adjust to new surroundings. Elderly clients may also worry about who will take care of a new pet if it outlives them. Offer these clients as much help and support as you can; they will need it.

> Be honest with your clients and don't surprise them.

Providing a way to preserve a memento of the pet for the client is a very caring gesture. A paw impression baked in clay, a lock of fur, or a favorite picture of the pet may be treasured for a long time. Offering urns or caskets for pets is also a good idea. Choices about burial and cremation should be discussed as soon as you know that death is imminent so the owner can think about the options and make a decision that he or she will feel good about later on.

When euthanasia is necessary, explain exactly how the procedure will be done and what to expect, both medically and emotionally. For example: "The veterinarian will give Spot an injection that is an overdose of anesthetic. He will fall asleep before the injection is completed, but it may take a few minutes for his heart and breathing to completely stop. During this time, you can pet or hold Spot and talk to him as much as you'd like." You might also warn the client that the pet may lose bladder or bowel contents and that its eyes will remain open.

If the death occurred at your hospital without euthanasia, many clients will want to view the body. They may want to do this with a team member, or they may prefer to be alone with the pet for a few minutes. They may also want other family members to have a chance to see the pet's body, so you may need to make arrangements to hold or even store the body for a short time. Clients will probably have questions about how or why the death occurred, so be sure the veterinarian or technician will be available to speak with them and to give them the correct answers.

Some clients become angry or blame the doctors or team for not being able to save their pets. This is a normal part of the grieving process and should be met with understanding and empathy, not defensiveness. Some clients blame themselves and have intense feelings of guilt and self-recrimination. Never say anything that implies that the pet's death was the owner's fault.

> Remember the Golden Rule.

For planned euthanasia, it may be best to have the client come in before the appointment to sign the paperwork and pay the bill. This separates the business activity from the loss of the pet, which can help the owner cope better. Payment matters could be settled the day before the scheduled euthanasia, or, if that is not possible, right before the procedure is performed. The point is that it is hard for most people to stop at the front desk and deal with payment just after they have watched their pet die. Owners also worry about falling apart in front of people at checkout or in the waiting room, and anything that simplifies what they have to do afterward is usually a relief to them. If you send the invoice to them, receiving it in the mail a few days later can reopen the painful wounds that were just beginning to heal. Your hospital may have policies for the timing of this, for example a two-week callback to mail the invoice, or you can ask each client what he or she would prefer.

Offer clients reading materials on pet loss and grief (see resources listed below). Team members who invest a little time in reading about grieving the loss of a pet can learn how to deal more comfortably with upset and grieving clients. Having a quiet room where you can discuss care and treatment for critically ill or injured animals, as well as perform euthanasia, can also be helpful.

Few things will endear a clinic to a client more than gentle, sensitive treatment during a pet's final hours or days. The more care you invest at this difficult time, the stronger the bond will be between your hospital and your community of clients.

RESOURCES

BOOKS FOR ADULTS

Anderson, Moira. 2007. *Coping with Sorrow on the Loss of Your Pet*, 3rd ed. Loveland, CO: Alpine Publications. Several sections from this book are available as brochures and handouts at www.pet-loss.net/handouts.shtml.

Argus Institute, Colorado State University. 2009. *What Now? Support for You and Your Companion Animal*. Lakewood, CO: AAHA Press.

DVM360, www.dvm360.com. This site has a euthanasia consent form and a euthanasia protocol. Look in "Practice Operations Forms" on the "Business Center" menu.

Lagoni, Laurel, Carolyn Butler, and Suzanne Hetts. 1994. *The Human-Animal Bond and Grief*. Philadelphia: W. B. Saunders.

Montgomery, Mary, and Herb Montgomery. 1993. *A Final Act of Caring: Ending the Life of an Animal Friend*. Minneapolis: Montgomery Press.

———. 2000. *Forever in Your Heart: Remembering My Pet's Life*. Minneapolis: Montgomery Press.

———. 1991. *Good-Bye My Friend: Grieving the Loss of a Pet*. Minneapolis: Montgomery Press.

Nakaya, Shannon Fujimoto. 2005. *Kindred Spirit, Kindred Care: Making Decisions on Behalf of Our Animal Companions*. Novato, CA: New World Library.

Quackenbush, Jamie, and Denise Graveline. 1985. *When Your Pet Dies: How to Cope with Your Feelings*. New York: Pocket Books.

Tousley, Marty. 1996. *Children and Pet Loss: A Guide for Helping*. Phoenix, AZ: Our Pals.

BOOKS FOR CHILDREN

Brown, Margaret Wise. 1979. *The Dead Bird*. New York: Dell.

Buscaglia, Leo. 1982. *The Fall of Freddie the Leaf*. New York: Holt, Rinehart and Winston.

Carrick, Carol. 1981. *The Accident*. New York: Houghton Mifflin.

Graeber, Charlotte. 1982. *Mustard*. New York: Macmillan.

Mellonie, B., and R. Ingpen. 1983. *Lifetimes*. New York: Bantam.

Morehead, Debby. 1996. *A Special Place for Charlie: A Child's Companion Through Pet Loss*. Broomfield, CO: Partners in Publishing.

Rogers, Fred. 1988. *When a Pet Dies*. New York: Putnam.

Viorst, Judith. 1987. *The Tenth Good Thing About Barney*. New York: Macmillan.

White, E. B. 1952. *Charlotte's Web*. New York: Harper Trophy Books.

Wilhelm, Hans. 1985. *I'll Always Love You*. New York: Crown.

OTHER RESOURCES

Allen, Moira Anderson. "Ten Tips on Coping with Pet Loss." Pet Loss Support Page, www.pet-loss.net/. Links on this page provide handouts and other resources.

American Animal Hospital Association (AAHA), www.aahanet.org/index.aspx. In addition to the book listed above by the Argus Institute entitled *What Now? Support for You and Your Companion Animal*, AAHA Press offers two brochures designed as client handouts: "When Your Pet Is Sick: A Resource for Pet Owners" and "The Loss of Your Pet: A Resource for Pet Owners."

American Veterinary Medical Association, Human Animal Bond Committee, www.avma.org. The AVMA has brochures entitled "Pet Loss: How Do I Know When It Is Time," "When Your Animal Dies," "Understanding Your Feelings of Loss," and "Equine Euthanasia: How Do I Know It Is Time?"

Argus Institute, Colorado State University, www.argusinstitute.colostate.edu/. The institute's website has sections on grief resources and pet hospice.

Grief Healing, www.GriefHealing.com. This website is run by bereavement counselor Marty Tousley and has resources on grief and healing, including discussion-group resources.

World by the Tail, www.veterinarywisdomforpetparents.com. This company offers handouts on pet loss and kits for making memorial paw impressions.

HEARTWORMS

Heartworms, the common name for the parasite species *Dirofilaria immitus*, are common and sometimes deadly, so clients need to know about them. Poor compliance in giving preventive medication to pets is often due to poor understanding of the severity and nature of the disease. According to an American Heartworm Society (AHS) survey conducted in 2008, 35 percent of owners who have their dogs seen annually by veterinarians fail to give their pets heartworm preventives. Only about one-third of the 1,000 dog owners surveyed knew that the disease was transmitted by mosquitoes. There are 1 million new canine heartworm cases in the United States every year because so many pets are unprotected.

The French heartworm, *Angiostrongylus vasorum*, and another related subcutaneous nematode found in Europe, called *Dirofilaria repens*, are expected to make their way into the United States eventually as a result of the mobile nature of today's society. *A. vasorum* has already been present in Newfoundland, Canada, since 2001. Soon we may need to educate clients about these parasite species as well.

There are 1 million new canine heartworm cases in the United States every year.

If you don't teach clients about heartworm disease, who will? It's absolutely the responsibility of veterinary team members to improve these statistics. However, don't expect clients to spend a lot of time learning about heartworm. People are busy, and you just won't have many clients who really want to delve into the life cycle of the parasite, the mosquitoes that carry it, or how the preventive medication works. Keep your message clear and simple.

Here's what you need to tell clients: "Heartworms are long worms the size and shape of spaghetti." (Eewwww! Feel free to make a face or grimace here: they truly are disgusting and doing so clearly communicates that to clients. Your expression will teach as effectively as your words.) "The larval form of the worm is carried by mosquitoes. If your dog [or cat] is bitten by a mosquito that is carrying larval heartworms, he [or she] could get this disease. The adult worms live in the dog's [or cat's] heart. This is not good for the heart: If your dog [or cat] gets heartworms, it could die. The disease is expensive to treat in dogs, and there is no effective treatment for cats. Your pet needs [note the word 'needs' here] to take this chewable, good-tasting tablet once a month so he [or she] doesn't get the disease if he [or she] is bitten by a mosquito that's carrying it."

The AHS survey revealed that 60 percent of those polled believed that the cost of treating heartworm disease in a dog was only about $250 and they thought it would be simple to treat—you prevent it with a pill, why wouldn't you treat it with one? They don't understand how lengthy, risky, and expensive treatment can be, or how serious the disease can be for the pet.

Pet owners, especially when the pet is a cat, may say, "But my pet never goes outside." Head them off at the pass. You can respond with, "Interestingly, about one-third of cats that get the disease stay strictly indoors. The few mosquitoes that come into your house are more than enough to carry the disease."

Then add, "The once-a-month pills have the added benefit of preventing the most common intestinal parasites as well. Did you know that 1 million to 3 million people, most of them children, pick up roundworms every year in the United States? Would you like to take the whole season's worth of pills today, or just the first two?" Don't offer the option of no pills at all!

Another common question clients ask concerns the need for heartworm testing even though the pet has been receiving heartworm-preventive medication. You can say, "It only takes one late or missed dose of preventive to open the door for infection, and regular testing ensures that we stop the disease early if that happens." Some clients are truly reliable in giving preventives on time every single month. Those are far outnumbered by the rest of the population. Most people occasionally slip up.

Don't present heartworm testing or prevention as an option unless you live in an area that sees very little of the disease. Routine, basic care should include parasite prevention. Some clients will still refuse, but, as usual, you are the advocate for the pet and must tell them what the pet needs to stay healthy.

If you have lots of heartworms in your area, hanging up a map and inserting red pins wherever a case was diagnosed can be a vivid educational tool for clients. Try to make the disease seem personal and topical: "We had another heartworm case just last week," "A cat died from heartworm at a clinic nearby just last month," and other similar statements help bring the disease close to home. It is common for people to assume that heartworm disease is rare and that the likelihood of their own pet contracting heartworms is low.

April is Heartworm Awareness Month. Use it as an opportunity to do something special. Heartworm disease can be fatal, yet it's almost 100 percent preventable. If we get the word out and focus on client compliance, there will be fewer unprotected pets.

Do something special during Heartworm Awareness Month in April. Heartworm disease can be fatal, yet it's almost 100 percent preventable. If we get the word out and focus on client compliance, there will be fewer unprotected pets.

If you have a DVD on heartworm disease, a heartworm model, or, best of all, an actual heartworm in a jar, make sure your clients (especially children) get to see it. These visual tools make a big impact and help to prevent clients from getting complacent and forgetting to give their pet the medication. Show a video about heartworm disease with a puppy or kitten visit to the hospital. The American Heartworm Society has client videos on their website. Few clients refuse the medication after seeing the large mass of squiggly worms on the video.

Unfortunately, when you've sold clients the medication, they still have to remember to give it. You might consider giving every client a calendar refrigerator magnet, with little red hearts drawn on the first or fifteenth of each month. This is not only helpful for the clients, but it's good advertising as well. You can also mark dates on the calendar magnet for flea product applications, dewormings, or surgery appointments. About two-thirds of pet owners forget to give at least one dose of monthly heartworm medication to their pets each year. Only a little over half of oral heartworm preventives sold are administered as directed. Moreover, when the pet owner forgets a dose, the average time before the medication is remembered and given again is 30 days. Approximately one-third of pet owners miss several doses, and about one-fifth forget so many that they give up and stop giving it altogether.

> *About two-thirds of pet owners forget to give at least one dose of monthly heartworm medication to their pets each year. . . . Approximately one-third of pet owners miss several doses, and about one-fifth forget so many that they give up and stop giving it altogether.*

If you or someone else on your team has the time to call or e-mail clients to remind them to pick up or give their pets their monthly pills, this can be a good practice builder. You don't need to call everybody, but forgetful seniors, busy parents, and clients with a family illness or crisis may appreciate this extra service. You can also help clients to set up automatic e-mail reminders for themselves, send out blast e-mails on the first and fifteenth of the month, or utilize text messaging or Tweets to do this. Technology should be used to make our hectic lives a little easier!

Many times when they forget to give a pet its monthly heartworm preventive medication, clients will call asking what to do. They should give the medicine to the pet as soon as they remember, but not double the dose to make up for the mistake. If a pet is temporarily ill, especially with vomiting or diarrhea, the client should wait until the pet is better before giving it the heartworm medication. The medication will be just as effective if it is given a week or so late. If it has been six weeks or more between monthly heartworm pills, there is an increased risk of the pet contracting the disease. However, the blood test checks for the previous year's infection, so it does no good to retest the blood of the dog until the following year. Heartworm disease is best treated early,

HEARTWORM ASSOCIATED RESPIRATORY DISEASE (HARD) IN CATS

The American Heartworm Society (AHS) and the American Association of Feline Practitioners (AAFP) are teaming up to get this urgent message out to cat owners. Their campaign messages center on five myths and misunderstandings about heartworm disease in cats.

Myth 1: It's a dog disease.
Heartworm disease affects cats differently than dogs, but the disease is equally serious in both.

Myth 2: It's a disease of outdoor cats.
It only takes one mosquito to infect a cat with heartworms. Because mosquitoes often manage to get indoors, both indoor and outdoor cats are at risk. In fact, one-third of affected cats never go outdoors.

Myth 3: It's a heart disease.
In cats, heartworms mainly affect the lungs, not the heart. Signs are often mistaken for asthma, allergic bronchitis, or other respiratory diseases. Coughing and wheezing, vomiting, and sudden death are the most common symptoms.

Myth 4: The cat must have one or more adult heartworms in the heart to become ill.
Heartworm larvae are actually the main cause of problems as they migrate through the lungs. Half of cats infected with heartworm larvae have damage to the small arteries that supply blood to the lungs.

Myth 5: Diagnosis is difficult.
Although falsely negative test results are common in cats, a positive test result is usually accurate. Cats should be tested if any of the common heartworm disease symptoms are present.

before extensive damage has occurred, so blood testing will continue to be needed on a regular basis to ensure a long, healthy life.

In addition, don't forget prevention for ferrets and cats! Heartworms parasitize many species, not just dogs.

RESOURCES

American Association of Feline Practitioners, www.catvets.com. AAFP's website has materials on HARD in cats.

American Heartworm Society, www.heartwormsociety.org. AHS posts the most current incidence map, content from prior Heartworm Society proceedings, survey and research data, and other useful information. It also has videos on canine and feline heartworm disease available for viewing online.

DVM360, Parasitology Center, http://veterinarycalendar.dvm360.com/avhc/Parasitology+Center/home/47731. Do a search from this page for "heartworm" for up-to-date information. Other articles and interactive quizzes can also be found on the site, including a sample heartworm reminder and "Feline Heartworm Q&A" under "Client Handouts" on the "Business Center" menu.

IDEXX Laboratories, www.idexx.com. IDEXX keeps heartworm statistics, too, and provides research articles online. Do a search from the home page for "heartworm" to access these.

INTESTINAL PARASITES

Intestinal parasites will be a frequent topic of conversation between you and your clients, so why not make it fun for your clients to learn about them? This is an opportunity to use educational displays, such as roundworms or tapeworms in formalin, or a graphically gross video. It's easy to make the topic rather interesting, and once they've learned about intestinal parasites in a fun way, people will take parasite problems more seriously. Unfortunately, because clients seldom actually see any worms in their pets' droppings, they usually underestimate the risk. They don't realize that most intestinal parasites are small and many are microscopic. Even large parasites such as roundworms are rarely seen in the stool; what we look for under the microscope is their tiny little eggs.

Clients tend to grimace at the thought of bringing in a stool sample. Who can blame them? Is there anything less fun for an owner to do with a pet than pick up some of its poop and bring it to the hospital? In fact, many clients never comply with stool-testing recommendations. How can we improve the odds that they will? A key thing to emphasize is that intestinal parasites can be a health threat to humans and animals. Protecting the pet means protecting the family, too.

Not warning clients about the hazards of intestinal worms to humans can become a liability problem for the practice, since roundworms, hookworms,

> **Be enthusiastic and creative!**

and Giardia are zoonotic (they affect humans too). Roundworm eggs are often deposited in the places where children play, and young children are more prone than others to putting their hands in their mouths and ingesting the eggs. This means that a toddler in the family or a visiting grandchild can contract roundworm—and if a client's pet wanders throughout the neighborhood, it means that the neighbors' children and grandchildren are put at risk as well. Over 1 million people—mostly children—contract roundworms every year in the United States, and more than 700 of them suffer blindness or permanent visual impairment as a result. Others suffer flulike symptoms of vomiting, diarrhea, and abdominal pain. Hookworm larvae can cause skin disease in humans, and Giardia can cause gastrointestinal disease.

These facts make it imperative that you educate your clients about intestinal parasites. Deworming, stool testing, and regular monthly parasite prevention are standard practice for dogs and cats from the very start, as most puppies and kittens already have parasites at birth or obtain them shortly thereafter (see "Intestinal Parasite Incidence in Puppies and Kittens" textbox). Everyone on your practice team should know what your clinic's parasite protocols are so that clients are given the same information by everyone and your educational materials support that approach.

When asked to collect stool samples year after year and visit after visit, most clients soon understand that it is a routine part of care. Some clients, however, are very resistant to checking for parasites because they don't want to pick up poop, or because they don't believe their pet is at risk. You may have

---

INTESTINAL PARASITE INCIDENCE IN PUPPIES AND KITTENS

About 95 percent of puppies and kittens are born with intestinal parasites or contract them shortly after birth. When female puppies are born, they have larval roundworms lying dormant in the walls of the uterus. When the puppy grows up and gets pregnant, these larvae migrate into her puppies to start the cycle over again. Encysted larvae are resistant to dewormers, so this cycle remains unbroken even with the modern dewormers now available.

more success with these clients if you can get a sample with a fecal loop during the office visit, or simply by practicing routine, scheduled dewormings. The latter is an especially good option for outdoor cats. Be flexible in your methods to improve compliance.

Clients are sometimes offended by the suggestion that their pets might have worms. They don't realize that all cats and dogs are susceptible. Dogs, especially, get worms because they have animal behaviors. Clients seem to forget that pets sniff and lick at disgusting things. They walk through stuff and then lick their feet. (Then they lick your face.) They hunt, kill, and eat birds, rodents, and rabbits. They eat rabbit poop and roll in raccoon droppings just for fun. Explain to clients that almost all wildlife carries parasites, and the parasite eggs survive for long periods of time in the grass or soil—waiting for their pet to come along and pick them up.

Because so many intestinal parasites are not worms at all but microscopic protozoa, it is best, in fact, never to use the word "worms" when discussing intestinal parasites with clients. In general, simpler is better, but you don't want to use incorrect layperson's terms either. Keep in mind that clients do not necessarily know the words "fecal," "feces," and even "stools." Sometimes clients are so busy trying to figure out what we are talking about that they miss half of what we say.

When talking about the importance of parasite control, describe the symptoms parasites can cause, and don't be afraid to be graphic. You might tell the client: "Symptoms of parasites include diarrhea, sometimes bloody, all over your carpet; vomit, sometimes with live worms in it, on your best bedspread; weight loss; poor hair coat; a potbellied look; poor appetite; poor performance in active sports such as hunting or agility; and illness of other family members because they picked up the parasites, too. It is wise to diagnose and treat your pet *before* any of these bad things happen." The clearer your description or imagery, the better the client will remember your recommendations.

You can also tell a story about a patient with parasites or even tell the client how much it would cost to deworm all of his or her pets if they pick something up. It can be very expensive, especially when the household includes several large dogs. If a pet is on year-round heartworm preventive provided by the family veterinarian, this cost can often be avoided. Most manufacturers guarantee their products and will pay for all or part of the treatment and recheck testing for any nematode parasites found up on fecal testing. If the client is getting the preventives online, these guarantees don't apply. This means you can use parasite treatment costs as a selling point for your hospital's heartworm products.

Be sure to recommend that clients pick up and dispose of animal feces regularly. The less poop lying around in the yard, the less chance the pet will

---

PARASITE FUN FACTS

- If a puppy vomits worms all over the kitchen floor, those are roundworms.
- Pregnant cats and dogs usually pass roundworms to their unborn offspring, even if the mother appears healthy.
- A single gram of feces from a pet with roundworms can contain 300,000 roundworm eggs!
- Hookworm larvae in the grass get inside a new host by penetrating through the skin of the feet.
- Because female whipworms lay eggs only periodically, a fecal sample may easily test negative for eggs. This makes the confirmation of a whipworm infection challenging. If symptoms are suggestive of whipworm presence, it's common to deworm for whipworms even if the fecal test is negative. On the days the female whipworms lay eggs, they lay between 4,000 and 8,000 eggs.
- Whipworm eggs are also not as buoyant as other parasite eggs, so they are more easily found using sugar solution and centrifugation to test the stool.
- The eggs of the whipworm *Trichuris suis* (found in swine) have been shown to survive in the environment for 11 years.
- Flea control is essential to control tapeworm infestation.
- Giardia can cause belching and flatulence in dogs.
- Giardia is the most common intestinal parasite of humans, but people usually have different strains than pets do.
- Just because a fecal sample tests negative doesn't mean the pet doesn't have worms. In one study, it was shown that 80 percent of puppies had *Toxocara* in their intestines even though only 20 percent tested positive on fecal exams.

become reinfested once any existing parasites have been dealt with. (See the section "Zoonotic Diseases" for more information.)

RESOURCES

Blagburn, Byron L. 2000. *Pfizer Atlas of Veterinary Clinical Parasitology*. New York: Pfizer. This book is nicely illustrated. Your Pfizer representative may be able to get it for you but you can also order it from booksellers.

Centers for Disease Control and Prevention (CDC), National Center for Infectious Diseases, Division of Parasitic Diseases, in cooperation with the American Association of Veterinary Parasitologists. "Guidelines for Veterinarians: Prevention of Zoonotic Transmission of Ascarids and Hookworms in Dogs and Cats." www.cdc.gov/ncidod/dpd/parasites/ascaris/prevention.htm. For more information from the CDC, see www.cdc.gov/healthypets. Useful CDC publications can be found at www.cdc.gov/parasites/animal.htm. They include "What Every Pet Owner Should Know About Roundworms and Hookworms" (www.cdc.gov/healthypets/Merial_CDCBroch_rsgWEB.pdf); "Toxoplasmosis: An Important Message for Women" (www.cdc.gov/parasites/toxoplasmosis/resources/toxowomen_2.2003.pdf); "Toxoplasmosis: An Important Message for Cat Owners" (www.cdc.gov/parasites/toxoplasmosis/resources/toxo_cat_owners_8-2004.pdf); and "Preventing Infections from Pets: A Guide for People with HIV Infection" (www.cdc.gov/hiv/resources/brochures/pets.htm).

Companion Animal Parasite Council, capcvet.org. This website and its companion site for pet owners, www.petsandparasites.org, have lots of good information, including parasite treatment and prevention protocols.

DVM360, www.dvm360.com. DVM360 has a parasite handout entitled "Parasites at a Glance." Look under "Client Handouts" on the "Business Center" menu.

"Get on Track with Parasite Compliance." 2010. *Veterinary Economics*, March 1.

Pfizer Atlas of Veterinary Clinical Parasitology. 1999. Wilmington, DE: Gloyd Group. Ask your Pfizer rep for a copy.

Stewart, Portia. 2009. "Extreme Makeover, Parasite Edition." *Veterinary Economics*, May 1.

JOINT DISEASE

Degenerative Joint Disease, or DJD, is one of the most common conditions we see in practice, affecting almost all dogs and cats eventually if they live long enough. Also known as osteoarthritis, OA, or just plain "arthritis," joint disease affects millions of pets. One in five dogs, regardless of age, is arthritic (20 percent of your canine caseload!), and 90 percent of cats over age 12 have visible arthritis on radiographs. The arthritis is painful in 20 percent of these older cats. (The older or heavier the cat, the more likely it is that it has arthritis pain.)

Because so many of the pets coming into your practice will have DJD, it is a topic you will spend a lot of time educating clients about. You will need to teach them not only how to treat it but how to recognize it in the first place. Pet owners are not always very savvy when it comes to recognizing pain in their pets, especially when the signs are subtle. It's up to us to teach them what to watch for.

As with many of the topics in this book, arthritis is a problem that will be diagnosed and discussed by the doctor when there are symptoms, but it is also a common subject discussed at wellness visits. The medications and supplements used to treat the disease are some of the most common products dispensed from veterinary pharmacies, so you will also have to communicate a lot of information on their use and safety. Pet owners generally have concerns

> **Be an advocate for the pet.**

about keeping their pets on any medication long-term, much less ones that can cause liver or kidney disorders. We need to be thorough and reassuring, knowing that clients feel more comfortable when they've received enough information.

Radiology has been the standard technique for diagnosing arthritis. Unfortunately, DJD doesn't become visible on radiographs until it is advanced, and there is little correlation between radiographic changes and the degree of lameness in the pet. Arthroscopy is becoming more common in dogs. Through "scoping" of joints, we are learning that many, many dogs have inflammation in their joints before they have lameness, changes on radiographs, or other symptoms.

> Listen to the client.

The history taken at the time of a senior examination or a lameness evaluation gives the veterinarian clues that arthritis may be present. When a pet is in pain from joint problems, usually the pet owner has already noticed changes in the pet's activity level. Based on the owner's and doctor's observation of these changes, the doctor will take a close look at the pet's range of motion and may do further testing.

The history taken from the client, in other words, is often going to determine whether a pet gets diagnosed and treated for this painful disease. And the client isn't going to come straight out and tell you the cat or dog is having pain unless he or she has been taught the signs to watch for. Getting a good history is as much about teaching the client what to look for as it is about obtaining information. Try using a form like the one at the end of this section.

Look for difficulty with rising, jumping, and moving in general in the pet. Ask the owner if the pet has difficulty with stairs, doesn't seek play anymore, or can't walk or run as fast or as far as before. Does the pet have a hard time jumping up onto furniture or into the car, or curling up in a bed or basket? Is the pet less active than it used to be, or seem depressed? Does it drag or scuff its toes, or have a poor appetite? Does it seek attention less than it used to? There may be lameness, or there may just be inactivity—the owner may notice that the pet is "slowing down." This is often because more than one area is sore—it may be difficult to limp if more than one leg is hurting. Inactivity is often a glaring sign of pain.

These questions are usually part of an exam history for older dogs. It's also important to realize that arthritis can be secondary to a defect or injury to a joint, so in some pets it can start very early in life. Hip dysplasia is often the underlying cause, but *luxating patellas* (i.e., kneecaps that slip out of place), elbow dysplasia, and leg deformities in some breeds also are predisposing problems. Orthopedic injuries that could lead to arthritis include a luxated hip, a torn anterior cruciate ligament (ACL) in the knee, or a fracture involving a joint. For all these reasons, incorporating questions about arthritis symptoms into the wellness history form for adult dogs will ensure no cases of DJD are missed.

Cats are more subtle with their symptoms, and owners often don't pick up on the fact that the cat isn't playing anymore or climbing on the scratching post. Spinal arthritis is common in cats but lower back pain can easily be missed. Cats with joint pain can exhibit "grumpiness" on handling, or they might seek seclusion. It is more difficult to perform range-of-motion tests on cats, so doctors rely even more on the owners' observations. This may require some careful probing. Lameness is not common in cats. But how high can the cat jump? Is it still climbing on its scratching post? Does it still enjoy playing? Is it grooming itself, or does it seem to hurt too much for the cat to twist or bend?

Litter-box avoidance is another tip-off that a cat may be having joint pain. This is common in elderly cats. It may hurt the cat to climb over the side or to squat to urinate or defecate, or the pan may be up- or downstairs that the cat can no longer navigate comfortably.

There are four stages of arthritis:

Stage 1: This stage refers to young animals predisposed to osteoarthritis due to conformation or injury.
Stage 2: Pets in this stage have current joint disease but little damage to joints and no symptoms.
Stage 3: Pets in Stage 3 have moderate damage and intermittent symptoms, often with decreased range of motion in the affected joints.
Stage 4: Severe damage and signs appear in this stage, such as atrophied muscles and restricted range of motion.

At Stage 4, the pet may resist, yelp, or even scream when the joint range of motion is tested. Cats will often attempt to bite with joint manipulation. The cartilage is mostly gone, so preserving it is no longer an option, and much of the pain stems from bone rubbing on bone. The owner may see difficulty rising, jumping onto furniture, going upstairs, or performing other activities. Lack of mobility is a life-threatening disease—dogs who can't get up or walk anymore (called "down dogs") are usually euthanized, as are cats who stop using the litter box. This is the stage we are trying to prevent by intervening early.

Joint disease is usually advanced before the pet is lame. Again, treatment should begin early in order to slow the progression of the disease and delay symptoms (and more expensive treatments) as long as possible. Our goal is to prevent or delay Stage 4.

It may be difficult to treat arthritis in the early stages because: (1) it's not evident there is a problem, and (2) owners are reluctant to believe their seemingly active, healthy pet has a serious problem simmering. Yet it is at this stage that the disease is the most preventable, and in fact early treatment can save years of suffering and a lot of money later on. So that's what we need to tell clients—"Even though you can't see it yet, your dog/cat is already in the early stages of arthritis. If we do nothing now, the pain and disability will be worse a few years down the road. Now is the time we can be the most successful at preserving the cartilage that lines the joints and decreasing the inflammation that eats that cartilage away."

Weight management is very important for arthritic pets. One study proved that overweight dogs develop symptoms of arthritis two years sooner than dogs of normal weight (Kealy et al. 2002; Lawler et al. 2005; Scarlett and Donaghue 1998). In addition, a weight loss of 10 to 15 percent results in improved clinical signs of arthritis, and a weight loss of as little as 5 to 10 percent improves mobility (Impellizeri et al. 2000). Keeping weight off is a key to preserving joint health for at-risk pets. (See the "Weight Control and Exercise for Pets" and "Pharmacy" sections. The latter covers teaching clients about drug risks and benefits, which will be applicable in arthritis cases.)

Arthritis is extremely common in both people and pets. The good news is that we are gaining a better understanding of the disease process all the time, and new drugs and therapies are greatly extending the quality of care we can provide. Teaching clients about this common and debilitating disease is not only a good investment of your time but can be life-changing for the affected pet.

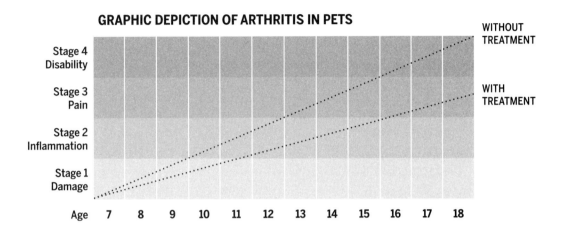

The above figure depicts the progression of arthritis that is treated and arthritis that is not. Arthritis is a chronic, progressive disease. We cannot cure it, and it will always gradually get worse. The goal is to slow its progress, trying to avoid having a pet ever get to Stage 4.

RESOURCES

American Association of Feline Practitioners, www.catvets.com. See the association's 2008 Pain Management Guidelines for cats, available at www.catvets.com/professionals/guidelines.

DVM360, www.dvm360.com. This website has a handout for clients entitled "Arthritis and Your Dog." Click on "Client Handouts" on the "Business Center" menu.

An Illustrated Guide to Orthopedic Conditions. 2005. Novartis Animal Health. Fort Collins, CO: Visible Productions. Ask your Novartis rep if you don't have one of these guides. They also have a helpful CD entitled *An Animated Guide to the Multimodal Management of Canine Osteoarthritis.*

North Carolina State University Comparative Pain Research Laboratory, www.ncsu.edu/project/cvm-pain/.

ARTHRITIS SCORE CARD

By filling out the following chart, you can help us to diagnose and stage arthritis in your pet. Some of these symptoms apply more to dogs, and some apply more to cats. Many apply to both. The more points your pet has, the more arthritis pain it is likely experiencing. Keeping track of symptoms on a daily basis can help you to monitor your pet's disease and also the response to treatments.

Grade your pet's symptoms according to the following scale:
(0) none, (1) mild, (2) moderate, or (3) severe.

Difficulty rising	0	1	2	3
Difficulty with stairs	0	1	2	3
Doesn't seek play anymore	0	1	2	3
Can't run as fast	0	1	2	3
Can't run as far	0	1	2	3
Can't walk as fast	0	1	2	3
Can't walk as far	0	1	2	3
Difficulty jumping up	0	1	2	3
Difficulty getting in and out of the litter box	0	1	2	3
Can't groom itself anymore	0	1	2	3
Can't curl up in a bed or basket	0	1	2	3
Inactive, depressed	0	1	2	3
Muscle atrophy	0	1	2	3
Drags or scuffs toes	0	1	2	3
Poor appetite	0	1	2	3
Doesn't seek attention	0	1	2	3

Total score

KITTENS AND PUPPIES

Your interaction with owners of new puppies and kittens lays the groundwork for all the health care those pets will need throughout their lives. The better those first few visits are, the better the care the puppy or kitten will receive later on. No one is more eager and excited to learn than the new puppy or kitten owner, so these first visits are prime times for teaching a lifetime of good pet-care habits.

Allow plenty of time on the first few visits to the clinic. Concentrate on building rapport with the client. Be sure you introduce yourself and other team members. Give out your business card and offer to answer the client's questions personally at any time. Using the business card format on a word processor program, you can print out as few or as many business cards as you like, and individual team members can have their own cards listing their areas of interest and expertise. This makes all team members appear more professional in the eyes of the client. If you have a brochure or newsletter, give it out as well.

> **Be enthusiastic and creative!**

These are the things you want new clients to know by the time they leave your office after the first visit:

- You care about their pet.
- Your office is clean, welcoming, and efficient.

- You can be the source of all their pet-care information—they should call whenever they have a question regarding any aspect of their pet's care.
- Pets that receive good veterinary care live much longer, healthier lives than those that don't.

Only when you have conveyed these vital messages can you concentrate on the other aspects of caring for the new pet.

Shyness has the highest heritability factor of all behaviors in dogs. That means that animals inherit a lot of their tendency to be shy or outgoing. "Socializing" a young pet with lots of human interaction helps to overcome shyness and teach it that interacting with human beings is a good thing. Research shows that in kittens, the socialization period is from three to seven weeks of age. The greater the number of people the kitten interacts with during this stage, the more social it will be both with its owners and with strangers, and the more likely it will become a "lap" cat.

> **Look and act professional.**

Make much of puppies and kittens every time they visit your hospital. Coo over them, give them treats, and ask the owners to bring them by "just for a visit." This helps accustom pets to the hospital environment and makes them better patients later on. It also wows clients, who will bask in your admiration of their new babies. Give away bandanas or kitty toys, take pictures of owners with their new friends, send them welcome cards, or call a few days after their first visit to see if they have any more questions.

After you've impressed the owner, focus on the pet. These are the things you want new puppies or kittens to know by the time they leave that day:

- Your clinic is a nice place where people will pet them, play with them, and care about them.
- No one will hurt them.
- You give them good treats to eat.

Pets can even get treats to eat while they're getting a vaccination. Handle the pet gently and calmly. An added benefit is that the less worried the owner is about the pet feeling stress or pain, the more the owner can concentrate on what you are trying to teach about pet care.

The veterinarians and team members should develop a standard protocol for all puppies and kittens during their vaccination series. This protocol lays out what owners should know at each stage of the pet's development and how these topics will be presented. A sample outline of such a protocol is provided below.

Consider giving every new client a three-ring binder with handouts appropriate for the pet's age and species. Go over the notebook page by page with the client. This ensures that no topics are forgotten. The notebook gives the owner a place to keep rabies certificates and other important papers. Add pages to the books every year on new breakthroughs that have occurred since the client's last visit, such as a new preventive medication or changes in vaccine schedules. For puppies and kittens, add extra handouts at each visit to cover the topics discussed at that visit.

> *Consider giving every new client a three-ring binder with handouts appropriate for the pet's age and species. Go over the notebook page by page with the client. . . . For puppies and kittens, add extra handouts at each visit to cover the topics discussed.*

Introduce the concept of breed-specific wellness during puppy and kitten visits. In dogs especially, breeds tend to have specific health problems that clients need to know about. Whether the pet is a bulldog, a Yorkie, a Doberman pinscher, or some other breed, there are specific issues that must be brought to the owner's attention. Different breeds have different temperaments, different disease risks, and even different nutritional needs.

It would be nice if every client called us before purchasing a new puppy for prepurchase counseling. In reality, only a small percentage of clients will seek advice from your team before the fact. But when they do, you should have materials or information at hand to help steer them toward a good choice for their family. Much heartbreak would be avoided if every client got an appropriate pet that fits his or her specific situation.

Most cats we see are not purebreds, so our focus with kittens is a little different. Risks are different for indoor and outdoor cats, so there are different educational needs for each. In addition, risks for contagious diseases play a bigger role with cats. When a kitten is at least 12 weeks old, it can be tested for feline leukemia virus (FeLV), feline immunodeficiency virus (FIV), and feline infectious peritonitis (FIP), and you can give the owner a "Fatal Feline Diseases" handout to read while he or she is waiting for test results. It can explain FeLV, FIV, and FIP; the tests being run that day; and the prices for FeLV and FIV vaccinations if you recommend them for this pet. It can also explain the risks cats incur when they go outdoors.

The second time the puppy or kitten is brought to the clinic, give the owner a toothpaste sample and a handout on dental care and demonstrate how to brush the pet's teeth. At the third puppy or kitten visit, discuss how to avoid and treat behavior problems, pre-anesthetic blood testing for surgery, microchipping, and, for dogs, the importance of obedience training. Also give the owner a handout outlining the care the pet will need before the next year's boosters. It can cover the importance of spaying and neutering, what to do about teething, the need for dental care as the pet grows older, nutritional needs and when to switch to adult food, when to return for heartworm testing, and the importance of the annual physical exam, especially in cats.

WARNING SIGNS

Puppies less than 14 weeks of age who growl warrant serious attention. They have very aggressive tendencies, and without exceptionally good training, may grow up to have serious behavior problems.

Discuss behavior issues early on, and let clients know that you are available to answer questions. Common issues that come up are house training, puppy play biting, jumping up on people, chewing, and submissive wetting. Most hospitals have team members who can address these sorts of problems.

The better the job we do teaching clients how to train a puppy, the less likely it will end up surrendered to a shelter for behavior problems later on.

Varied and complex environments lead to increased brain development. Pet shop or puppy mill puppies and kittens often have a lack of neurological development as a result of lack of stimulus. Breeders should expose puppies and kittens to varied stimuli—such as different people, floor surfaces, and noises. The critical period for this is five to seven weeks of age, before most new owners acquire their pets.

> **Be an advocate for the pet.**

Offer puppy-training classes and a kitten kindergarten session that covers scratching posts, preventing litter-box avoidance, dealing with scratching and biting, normal play behavior, and socialization.

Sometimes an older cat comes in, presented for weight loss, who hasn't been to a veterinarian since it was spayed or neutered years before. Now it has hyperthyroidism and hypertension on top of chronic kidney disease and a mouth full of infected teeth. The owner becomes so overwhelmed at how much needs to be done that many times he or she ends up euthanizing the cat. If we had been seeing the cat all along, we would have taken care of the teeth before the bacteria caused kidney damage. We could have treated the hyperthyroidism and hypertension early as they arose and the cat would have lived three or four more years. This all-too-common scenario could be avoided in many cases if we only did a better job of explaining the importance of health care early on. Develop scripts to use to emphasize this. For example, "Pets that receive good health care throughout their lives live years longer than pets that don't." If you know the messages you need to get across at each stage of the pet's life and plan how you are going to do that, you are more likely to succeed in communicating them.

Sadly, our culture does not value cats as highly as dogs. We all have those clients who bring their dogs in faithfully every year but who will not let us see their cats. It's difficult to change people's attitudes, but we can certainly do our best to teach people what cats need and deserve to have in the way of care. The American Association of Feline Practitioners (AAFP) Feline Handling

EXAMPLE OF A PUPPY PROTOCOL

First Visit: 40–50 minutes with doctor

- Distemper-Hepatitis-Parainfluenza-Parvovirus (DHPP), unless recently vaccinated
- Bordetella, 1 of 2
- Fecal centrifugation, deworm as needed and according to Centers for Disease Control and Prevention (CDC) and Companion Animal Parasite Council (CAPC) guidelines
- Office visit, new patient/Humane Society exam
- Notebook and puppy kit
- Bandana

Complete physical exam with report card. Discuss vaccines; parasites: housebreaking, socialization; getting accustomed to ears, toes, and mouth being handled. Go over obedience training and importance of spaying or neutering. Discuss diet. Discuss bathing and grooming. Review entire puppy notebook. Start on heartworm meds and flea control if warm weather.

Second Visit: 30–40 minutes with technician

- Distemper-Hepatitis-Leptospirosis-Parainfluenza-Parvovirus (DHLPP), unless recently vaccinated
- Bordetella, 2 of 2
- Office visit, well patient exam by technician
- Sample toothpaste

Discuss and demonstrate dental care. Discuss any problems with housebreaking or behavior. Recheck any problems from first visit (ear mites, skin, etc.). Dispense additional heartworm and flea meds, if necessary. Make sure puppy is growing normally. Discuss diet again, if necessary.

Third Visit: 30 minutes with technician

- DHLPP
- Office visit with technician

- View heartworm DVD
- Bandana

No physical exam unless puppy is having problems. (Recheck any prior problems again.) Discuss Lyme disease vaccine, if needed. Ask how tooth brushing is going. Review behavior again. Teach nail trimming. Dispense more heartworm and flea meds, if necessary. Review nutrition and amount being fed. Recheck fecal centrifugation and perform Giardia SNAP if not already done.

Fourth Visit: 30 minutes with doctor
- Rabies vaccination by doctor
- Lyme disease vaccination, if needed
- Bandana
- Exam for proper dental development and common puppy problems such as pyoderma and vaginitis
- Discuss breed-specific problems that are likely to occur during puppyhood, including any extra recommended testing

If this is the pet's last vaccination visit, give the client a handout covering health-care issues he or she will need to be aware of from this point on, such as the need for annual heartworm testing and intestinal parasite screening, and go over it together. Give the client brochures on pre-anesthetic blood testing and microchipping. Review teething, chew toys, and tooth brushing. Ask about housebreaking. Give heartworm or flea meds, if needed. Review the need for obedience training. Go over health risks for puppies of this breed. (Untrained dogs are five times more likely to be surrendered to a humane society than trained dogs.)

Fifth Visit (Plus): 20 minutes with both doctor and technician
- Second Lyme disease vaccination
- Bandana
- Give client "Pre-anesthetic Blood Testing" brochure
- Go over "What's Next" handout

Note: Protocols will vary with geographic location and local disease incidence.

EXAMPLE OF A KITTEN PROTOCOL

First Visit: 40 minutes with doctor

- Feline Viral Rhinotracheitis-Calicivirus-Chlamydia-Panleukopenia vaccination (FVRCCP), unless recently vaccinated
- Fecal centrifugation, dispense dewormers as needed according to Centers for Disease Control and Prevention (CDC) and Companion Animal Parasite Council (CAPC) recommendations
- Office visit, new patient/Humane Society exam
- Notebook, report card
- Pet kit

Complete physical exam. Discuss all topics in notebook, including vaccines, parasites, feline leukemia (FeLV) and feline immunodeficiency virus (FIV), feline lower urinary tract disease (FLUTD) symptoms, spaying and neutering, and declawing. Discuss diet, behavior, and litter-box usage. Discuss bathing and grooming, handling of feet, mouth, and ears. Dispense heartworm and flea meds, if needed.

Second Visit: 30 minutes with technician

- FVRCCP
- Office visit, well patient exam
- Sample toothpaste
- Report card

Discuss and demonstrate dental care. Recheck any problems from first visit (ear mites, fleas, etc.). Discuss any behavior problems. Discuss diet again, if necessary. Dispense flea and heartworm meds, if needed.

Third Visit: 30 minutes with doctor or technician

- FeLV and FIV testing and information, results sheet
- FVRCCP and FeLV vaccines
- View heartworm DVD while blood test is being done

No physical exam unless problems are present. Recheck any prior problems and teach nail trimming. Discuss FIV vaccine if kitten goes outside. Discuss spaying and neutering and declawing information. Recheck fecal sample if not already done. Dispense heartworm or flea meds, if needed.

Fourth Visit: 20 minutes with doctor
- Rabies shot
- Second FeLV vaccine

Give client "What's Next" handout on upcoming concerns and brochures on pre-anesthetic blood testing and microchipping. Review nutrition, spaying and neutering, and declawing information. Review the need for annual exams and vaccines even if cat is always indoors. Dispense heartworm or flea meds, if needed. Emphasize the importance of regular checkups, stool checks, and vaccinations, even for indoor cats.

Note: Protocols will vary with geographic location and local disease incidence.

Guidelines can help. We can also demonstrate every day in the way we handle cats and kittens that we know that they are important and valuable.

Clients who have acquired a new puppy or kitten are usually the ones who are most willing to learn about care for their pet. Even if their good intentions eventually fade away, at these first visits you will have the best chance you'll ever have to turn them into good pet owners. Spread the vaccines out over as many visits as possible to maximize the time available to teach clients what they need to know about caring for their new friend.

A comprehensive program for new pets is vital to maximizing your hospital's impact on the growth and development of its most important new patients. Done well, this type of program will create loyal, bonded clients who will return to your practice for the duration of the pet's life, who will tell others about your practice, and who will trust you to guide them in their pet-care decisions for many years to come.

RESOURCES

American Animal Hospital Association. Canine Vaccine Guidelines Revised, http://secure.aahanet.org/eweb/dynamicpage.aspx?site=resources&webcode=CanineVaccineGuidelines.

American Association of Feline Practitioners, www.catvets.com. See "2010 Feline Life Stage Guidelines, www.catvets.com/professionals/guidelines/publications/?Id=425; and "Respectful Handling of Cats to Prevent Fear and Pain," www.catvets.com/uploads/PDF/Nov2009HandlingCats.pdf. "Feline Handling Techniques" will be released in 2011; see www.catvets.com/professionals/guidelines/publications/ for updates. See also "Creating a Cat Friendly Practice" at www.fabcats.org/catfriendlypractice/guides.html.

Boss, Nan. 2003. *The Client Education Notebook: Customized Client Education Materials to Use in Your Own Practice.* Lincoln, NE: AVLS-PetCom. This is my complete set of handouts for all routine pet care, which I developed for use in my own hospital.

DVM360, www.dvm360.com. This site lists several behavior tools appropriate for puppy and kitten visits. Under the "Business Center" menu, choose "Patient Care Forms." Look for "Pre-adoption Counseling Resources," "Behavior Questionnaire," "Behavior Assessment Checklist," and "Behavior History Form." Under "Client Handouts" you'll find "Overcoming Common Behavior Problems in Kittens," "Teaching Your New Puppy the Right Way to Play," "Why Punishment Fails; What Works Better," and "How to Create Low-Stress Veterinary Visits for Cats."

Gough, Alex, and Alison Thomas. 2004. *Breed Predispositions to Disease in Dogs and Cats.* Oxford: Blackwell.

Hart, Benjamin L., and Lynette A. Hart. 1987. *The Perfect Puppy.* New York: W. H. Freeman.

James and Kenneth Publishers, www.jamesandkenneth.com/. This publisher offers books, videotapes, and behavior booklets by Dr. Ian Dunbar that work well for puppy classes. These are great materials to use in developing puppy classes, especially the *SIRIUS® Puppy Training* DVD and Doctor Dunbar's 2003 *Good Little Dog* book.

Kilcommons, Brian, and Sarah Wilson. 1999. *Paws to Consider: Choosing the Right Dog for You and Your Family.* New York: Warner Books.

McConnell, Patricia B. 1996. *Dog's Best Friend's Beginning Family Dog Training.* Black Earth, WI: Dog's Best Friend.

VetThink, www.vetthinkinc.com. This company publishes the Genesis Breed-Specific Health Care Wellness Books, a series of booklets and handouts on each of 75 different breeds to give to clients. It also offers breed-specific electronic newsletters. Each breed booklet for clients includes a chart of services recommended at different ages specific to the needs of that breed. This includes screening for genetic diseases at the time of spaying or neutering.

Walkowicz, Chris. 1996. *The Perfect Match: A Buyer's Guide to Dogs*. New York: Howell Book House.

White, Linda M. 2009. *First Steps with Puppies and Kittens: A Practice-Team Approach to Behavior*. Lakewood, CO: AAHA Press.

Whitehead, Sarah. 2010. *Adolescent Dog Survival Guide*. Wenatchee, WA: Dogwise.

LABORATORY TESTING

In the past, even owners of critically ill pets had to wait hours or days for a diagnosis until their pets' blood test results came back from the laboratory. With the advent of inexpensive test kits and benchtop lab equipment, same-day or same-hour test results are now the standard of care in most veterinary hospitals. This technology has revolutionized the practice of medicine, allowing pre-anesthetic and wellness blood testing, quick screening for diseases such as feline leukemia and parvovirus, and a high level of care for critically ill patients. Laboratory testing likely accounts for 15 to 20 percent of the income of your practice.

In 1960, the average dog lived to be only six years old. Today the average dog lives almost twice that long, and most indoor cats live to be 15 or more years old. Because so many cats and dogs are living longer, there is an increasingly large population of senior pets. Keeping these older animals happy, healthy, and pain-free and maximizing their life expectancy have created a large demand for services such as senior blood work and screening electrocardiograms (ECGs).

Pets, just like people, need screening tests for common diseases as they grow older. Kidney disease, heart disease, and thyroid abnormalities become increasingly common as dogs and cats age—and because they age more quickly than humans, testing is usually needed at least once a year.

Clients expect a high level of technology in medical care. They aren't shocked to be asked about blood screening or preoperative ECGs. Many clients not only expect these things but will go elsewhere if your clinic does not offer them. New screening tests are available now as well, including blood tests for cancer and heart disease markers, DNA tests for genetic disorders, and new enzyme-linked immunosorbant assay (ELISA) and polymerase chain reaction (PCR) tests for disease diagnosis. As prices come down and availability increases, we will be able to incorporate even more tests into our repertoire.

As a team you can implement new ways to use your lab equipment to help your patients. A complete blood count (CBC) performed when a pet is young and healthy can give you a baseline. Knowing what a pet's normal hematocrit is helps us to determine whether it is anemic or dehydrated later on when it is showing signs of illness. Knowing a dog's normal white blood cell count (WBC) helps us to know whether an infection is brewing later on.

Your clinic can also use diagnostic testing to help specific breeds and to keep on top of changes at specific stages of pets' lives. Breeds such as boxers, Doberman pinschers, and English cocker spaniels, for example, are prone to cardiomyopathy, an often deadly form of heart disease. An ECG screen performed each year can detect an abnormal heart rhythm when the dog is still in the early stages of the disease—when it can be helped the most. Annual urine testing for older patients allows early detection of diabetes, bladder stones, and kidney disease.

These advances mean that you must spend more time with clients promoting these lab tests and explaining the results. All of this testing can be expensive, so clients need to feel they are getting value for their money. Involve the client in the decision-making process and explain what the tests will tell the doctor.

Most clinics have found that how wellness testing is presented is important. Offer pre-anesthetic, breed-specific, and senior testing with enthusiasm. These tests allow for detection of diseases in their earliest stages, before they result in complications or overt signs of illness. If pre-anesthetic testing reveals a problem, adjustment of the anesthetic protocol or fluid therapy during the procedure may be warranted. If kidney, liver, or thyroid disease is detected, early treatment can be lifesaving. You can tell the client, "We are so excited about being able to offer this high level of testing for our patients. It can save the life of your pet and we'll have results back in just 30 minutes. Would you prefer the regular screen, which tests for 12 different things and can be used as a baseline for the rest of your pet's life, or the mini-screen, which gives us three tests?" This script is an example of a technique that offers the client two "yes" options instead of a "yes" and a "no." You'll have to explain the pluses and minuses of both options. The client can say no, but when the options are presented in this way, as the standard of care rather than the exception, most clients will choose one or the other test instead of refusing both.

> **Be enthusiastic and creative.**

Use terms clients understand and that aren't frightening to them. Clients prefer to hear the word "senior" versus "geriatric," for example, because "geriatric" makes them think of nursing homes and dying. Pet owners don't want to think of their pets as "old." It can also be very effective to correlate the pet's age to human age: "If Fluffy were a person, she would be over 50 now, so we need to look more closely for problems that start to occur at this age." Clients like to feel special and they are pleased when you seem to know a lot about their specific breed of dog or cat, so use that method as applicable. Don't just say, for example, "Max needs a blood test screening today." Instead, show your understanding of Max and his needs by saying, "Dobermans like Max are particularly prone to hepatitis, a form of liver disease, so it's especially important to do blood test screening regularly."

Clients are much more likely to agree to laboratory testing if they fully understand what the tests are and why they are important.

A key point is that clients are much more likely to agree to laboratory testing if they fully understand what the tests are and why they are important. Explain why the doctor want to perform the tests and what the results will mean. For example, when discussing a CBC, you need to say something like "This is a complete blood count. It tells us how many and what kinds of white blood cells are circulating in the blood right now, and whether your pet is anemic or has enough platelets." For a chemistry panel, you might say, "This test tells us how well the kidneys and the liver are functioning." If the pet is ill, say, "Spot may not be feeling well because of a liver or kidney problem we can't see from the outside. These tests will help us to find out what's wrong." Use easy-to-understand language and tie the tests to human health, if possible.

Team members need to mention wellness testing to clients early and often. With each visit of middle-aged pets approaching senior status, mention the need for future senior testing. Handouts, videos, or newsletter articles can also help you offer and promote laboratory services. The more times clients are exposed to the concepts behind lab testing recommendations, the more likely they are to have them done. With each mention, you are showing your confidence in the fact that the screenings are necessary.

Your hospital will only be successful at recommending laboratory services if every team member understands the tests and agrees that they are important for health care in the pets that come to your clinic. For example, anyone who thinks pre-anesthetic blood tests are a waste of time and money won't sell them to clients effectively. It can't be emphasized enough that practicing good medicine requires the support and backing of the entire hospital team. It is likely that more than one team member will be presenting the clients with the lab testing options, and everyone needs to be good at it.

> Be an advocate for the pet.

Each member of the team must learn to avoid saying wishy-washy things like "We recommend pre-anesthetic blood testing, but it's an option and you don't have to do it if you don't want to." You must be an advocate for the pet and you must sound confident about the value of tests you are recommending. Your job is to think about what is best for the health and comfort of the animal. If your clinic's doctors believe that anesthesia is not safe without blood testing done first, then you must say to the client, "Buffy needs to have pre-anesthetic blood testing today before surgery." Clients can still decline services they don't want or can't afford, but if you believe in good care, offer good care, not mediocre care.

When test results come back, the client will be pleased to hear that everything looks normal. Don't feel bad about saying the results were okay! The client doesn't want to hear that Spot has a dreadful disease; he or she wants to hear that Spot is going to live a long time. Be sure to tell the client all the things that weren't wrong with Spot: "Ms. Jones, I have good news. Spot's test results showed no liver or kidney abnormalities, no anemia, and no diabetes." Be sure to offer a printout or copy of the test results, with an explanation of their meaning.

Write it down!

Be enthusiastic, positive, and bold when advising laboratory testing for your patients. It's one of the best ways to help them live long and happy lives.

The following forms are some tools you can use for both offering clients wellness laboratory testing and for giving them the results. If you use them in your hospital they should be customized to fit protocols and the specific tests that are run.

RESOURCES

American Association of Feline Practitioners, www.catvets.com. See "Friends for Life: Caring for Your Older Cat," www.catvets.com/healthtopics/wellness/?Id=422.

Antech Laboratories, www.antechdiagnostics.com. Statistics for positive test results at various ages are on the "Continuing Education" page, and there is also some good information in Antech's newsletters. Click the "Have You Heard" dropdown menu and choose "Newsletters."

DVM360, www.dvm360.com. DVM360 lists several items to help with laboratory screening programs. Under the "Business Center" menu, choose "Client Handouts." Look for "Understanding Your Pet's Blood Work," "Facts About Long-Term Care" (about medication monitoring), and "Client Education Handout on Blood Testing."

Idexx Laboratories, www.idexx.com. Click the "Education" tab to learn about Idexx's online continuing education offerings.

"I Want to Test Your Pet's Blood." 2006. *Veterinary Economics*, December 1.

McClain, Laura. 2008. "Talking to Clients About Preanesthetic Testing." *Veterinary Economics*, July 1.

Metzger, Fred, and Cynthia Wutchiett. 2006. "10 Reasons to Test In-House." *Veterinary Economics*, November 1.

Wutchiett Tumblin and Associates. 2010. *Benchmarks 2009: A Study of Well-Managed Practices*. Columbus, OH: Wutchiett Tumblin and Associates, with *Veterinary Economics*.

BASELINE CBC

As part of your dog's routine health program, we recommend that a CBC be done with your pet's first annual vaccination or heartworm test. A CBC, or complete blood count, measures the number of each kind of cell found in the blood, including red and white blood cells and platelets.

"Normal" blood counts vary substantially from one dog to another. A white blood cell count of 14,000, for example, may mean an infection for a dog whose usual count is 7,000. For another dog, 14,000 may be perfectly okay.

Doing a CBC when your dog is young and healthy gives us a baseline with which to compare later results for the rest of your dog's life. If your pet becomes ill, it will then be much easier to interpret the blood test results and make an accurate diagnosis of his or her condition.

The cost of doing the CBC is $ .... Please let us know whether or not you wish to have a CBC test done for your pet today.

ECG SCREENING FOR BOXERS AND DOBERMAN PINSCHERS

Boxers, English cocker spaniels, Doberman pinschers, and many other breeds are prone to a heart condition called cardiomyopathy. Up to half of all dogs of these three breeds will eventually develop the disease. Cardiomyopathy thins and deteriorates the heart muscle, eventually leading to heart failure.

Cardiomyopathy can start as early as 6 months of age, or as late as 15 years, but most affected dogs start developing symptoms at 6 to 8 years of age. By the time symptoms develop, the heart is already severely damaged. Life expectancy at this stage is usually short—months to a year or two.

Diagnosing the disease early, and starting the affected pet on heart medication, can prolong life expectancy for these dogs by one to three years. Echocardiography is the most accurate way to diagnose the disease, but many dogs will start to show abnormalities on an ECG in the early stages of the disease.

A simple ECG strip, done once a year for less than $ .... , is a screening test for cardiomyopathy that should be done annually for all boxers, English cocker spaniels, and Doberman pinschers over one year of age, along with their annual vaccinations.

WELLNESS PROGRAM TEST RESULTS

Interpretation of test results is complicated. Some results are clear-cut and others difficult to interpret. Further testing, or retesting at a later date, may be necessary to diagnose a problem. Changes can occur quickly as pets age or become ill. We recommend blood testing at least once a year as your pet grows older.

NAME OF TEST	RESULT	NORMAL RANGE	EXPLANATION
BUN Creatinine			BUN and creatinine levels increase with kidney disease. BUN can also go up from stress, fever, or dehydration.
Alkaline Phosphatase ALT AST CK			These are enzymes from inside cells. When cells are damaged, enzymes leak out and show up in the blood. Alkaline phosphatase comes from many different cells. ALT and AST are liver enzymes. CK is a muscle enzyme.
Glucose			High blood sugar can mean diabetes. Stress can also cause elevated glucose, especially in cats.
Total Protein Albumin Protein Globulin Protein Albumin/Globulin Ratio			Protein levels are elevated with dehydration and can go up or down with cancer, liver, or intestinal disease. Albumin is made by the liver. Globulins make up antibodies that fight disease. We also look at the ratio between the two proteins.
Cholesterol			Cholesterol may become elevated with liver diseases, hypothyroidism, or adrenal problems.
Total Bilirubin			Bilirubin may be elevated with liver disease and some forms of anemia.
Sodium Potassium Calcium Phosphorus Chloride CO_2			The electrolytes, or salts in the bloodstream, tell us about dehydration, hormone imbalances, toxemia, and many other problems. They go up or down with various diseases.
T4			This is a thyroid hormone. Older cats frequently have too much T4 (hyperthyroidism) and dogs frequently have too little (hypothyroidism).

CBC RESULTS (NOT ALL PANELS INCLUDE A CBC)

White Blood Cell Count: White blood cells fight infections. High numbers usually mean infection is present. Bacteria, viruses, fungi, parasites, and allergies may all cause high white blood cell counts. There are five different types of white blood cells. Elevations of different types indicate the type and severity of infection. Low white blood cell counts may indicate life-threatening viral infections, cancer, or toxicity.

Red Blood Cell Count: Red blood cells are produced by bone marrow. Anemia, or low red blood cell count, results from loss of red blood cells, as with hemorrhage (bleeding), or from destruction of red blood cells from parasites or toxins. Red blood cells can also be destroyed by the body's own immune system. Decreased production of red blood cells usually means bone marrow disease, and a bone marrow biopsy is indicated.

Hemoglobin and Hematocrit: These values indicate the oxygen-carrying ability of your pet's blood and the degree of blood loss. Elevation of the hematocrit indicates dehydration.

A. Your pet passed! All tests were normal.

B. Your pet passed, but tests indicate some areas of concern.

C. Tests indicate major organ function disorders and need immediate attention!

The .... was ☐ High ☐ Low, indicating ....

The .... was ☐ High ☐ Low, indicating ....

The .... was ☐ High ☐ Low, indicating ....

The .... was ☐ High ☐ Low, indicating ....

We will need to test your pet again for .... in ....

SENIOR WELLNESS TESTING FOR YOUR HEALTHY OLDER PET

Pets age much more rapidly than humans. With the aging process, changes occur in the function of the body. Some of these changes can be seen from the outside: weight gain or loss, stiffness, dull hair coat, and loss of sight or hearing. Some changes, however, occur internally and cannot be detected without laboratory testing. Unfortunately, by the time symptoms of illness can be seen—in kidney or liver disease, for example—organ damage is already in the advanced stages.

To detect organ damage in its early stages, when it can be treated most successfully, we recommend annual blood and urine testing as part of your pet's yearly physical examination once he or she is more than seven to nine years of age. This testing can also be used as a baseline for comparison in the event of future illness, allowing us to identify changes and assist in a faster, more accurate diagnosis. You will receive a copy of the test results for your records.

Test results serve double duty by providing information before surgery or dental procedures, allowing for safer anesthesia.

Early detection can mean a longer, healthier life for your pet. Please let us know your decision on this important testing for your pet by checking off the box that is right for your pet. The doctor will go over the testing choices with you.

.... **Basic Screen:** This chemistry and electrolyte screen gives us information on kidney and liver function and blood sugar level. This is the minimum testing necessary for safe anesthesia in older pets.

The cost of this test is $ ....

.... **Silver Screen:** This screen includes the chemistry and electrolyte levels described above as well as thyroid testing. Thyroid testing is especially important for pets over age 12 or those showing signs of aging or illness, such as weight gain or loss, dry skin, and heart murmurs.

The cost of this test is $ ....

Because of the age, breed, or health status of your pet, the doctor has recommended additional testing. These extra tests are:

ECG, $ ....

Complete blood count (CBC), $ ....

Spinal/hip X-rays, $ ....

Chest X-rays, $ ....

Urinalysis, $ ....

Urine protein:creatinine ratio (UPC) for kidney disease, $ ....

Intraocular pressure (glaucoma screening), $ ....

Schirmer tear test, to screen for dry eyes, $ ....

Cancer screening for ...., $ ....

DNA testing for ...., $ ....

Problems to Watch For

Obesity	Liver Disease	Rear Leg Weakness
Arthritis	Tooth/Gum Disease	Poor Hair Coat
Kidney Disease	Diabetes	Impaired Senses (hearing, sight, smell)
Heart Disease	Cancer	Memory Loss (loss of habits)

If you do not want any screening tests and would like to waive your animal's rights to these needed procedures, please indicate by signing below.

Agent authorized to waive care:

....
SIGNATURE   **DATE**

MONEY MATTERS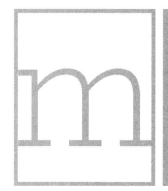

Many times, team members find talking about money with clients to be difficult. Team members and clients alike can get defensive, resulting in miscommunication and hurt feelings. When dealing with financial matters, clear communication and good documentation are vital to avoiding disputes. Office policies about payment plans and deposits should be crystal clear. If yours aren't, the practice leaders should sit down and devise some rules to avoid repeating the same mistakes and problems and reduce confusion.

Keep in mind that veterinarians and team members deserve to be paid good salaries and to have health insurance, vacations, and other benefits. Your building and equipment need to stay up-to-date. Costs for insurance, utilities, rent or mortgage, advertising, and every other thing in the budget go up every year. What veterinary teams do is valuable to clients—you deserve to be paid for your time, knowledge, and effort. If you want to be paid appropriately and get a raise next year, you have to get that money from your clients. Never be embarrassed or ashamed to ask for the money a client owes. That money covers both your paycheck and every other expense of the clinic.

Making sure money matters are handled properly begins as soon as clients come into your clinic. It continues as your team prepares an estimate or healthcare plan for needed services, explains that estimate, discusses payment options, and presents the invoice to the client after the services are rendered. If any part of this process is overlooked, the clinic may end up with nonpaying clients, and this makes it difficult to stay profitable and keep up with expenses.

This section will look at each step of this process. It will help your team devise policies for handling these very important issues by looking at five key money topics: pet insurance, new clients, estimates, presenting invoices, and doing pro bono work.

PET INSURANCE

Third-party payment services such as CareCredit, along with pet insurance plans, will often encourage or allow clients to afford services they could not easily manage otherwise. In the case of insurance, the client has to have the plan in place before an injury or illness will be covered, so our job is to make sure clients know about these programs early on. Emergency care for a serious problem costs serious money nowadays. Clients who are unprepared for the sudden expense are often forced to make a decision to euthanize their pet.

> Repetition is key.

We need to educate clients about pet insurance at their first wellness visit and repeat the message several times. I generally tell my clients: "If your dog breaks his leg and it would cost several thousand dollars to repair it, and you could afford to do so, you probably don't need pet insurance. If spending that money would severely impact your finances, then pet insurance is probably a really good idea." You'll need to direct clients toward a good source of information about pet insurance, either by recommending specific companies or steering them to a website comparing the options. (You can find more information at PetInsuranceReview.com. The American Animal Hospital Association [AAHA] also has a program called "Seal of Acceptance" that you can read about at www.aahanet.org/resources/whitepapers.aspx.)

NEW CLIENTS

When a new client comes in for the first appointment, be sure the forms he or she fills out ask how the bill will be paid. Check this "new client" form before escorting the client to the exam room. If the payment method is not filled out, ask the client directly how he or she will be paying the bill. The time to find out that the client has no money is before the patient is treated, not after.

First-time clients, or clients who have only been in a few times for minor services, should also be required to leave a large deposit for services (based on an accurate estimate) before they leave their pets for a workup or surgery. The majority of nonpaying clients are first-time clients. Some nonpaying clients have a long history of nonpayment or bounced checks elsewhere. A quick Internet search sometimes saves you from being the next victim.

If a client has been coming to your practice for 5 or 10 years and had never gotten behind on his or her account, it's less likely he or she will become a nonpayer. For these people, you still must do an estimate for anything beyond a normal office visit, but you can rest assured that the clinic probably won't be left footing the bill.

GIVING ESTIMATES

First of all, although we commonly refer to them as "estimates," in many practices it's customary to refer to them as "health-care plans." The reasoning for this is that we get estimates for car or appliance repair and we would rather clients not think of health care for their pets in the same way.

If your practice is one of these, you can substitute "health-care plan" wherever you see the word "estimate."

Clients have the right to know what they are spending and what they will get for their money. Give accurate estimates and update clients when the charges increase. Clients are much happier to pay their bills if they are forewarned

> **Remember the Golden Rule.**

about how much they will be. Your customers have the right to know what services they are receiving for their pets and what other care alternatives exist. This is true not just for in-hospital care but for outpatient visits as well. My teams prepare an estimate for almost every appointment they see. Even for routine visits, by the time we perform wellness screening, heartworm testing, a fecal exam, and 12 months of heartworm and flea preventives, it adds up to a hefty total, especially if the owner has multiple pets. If your practice doesn't have a process set up for providing estimates, come up with some ideas for formalizing this and share them with the practice leadership.

Providing both short- and long-term, accurate prognoses is part of the equation in estimating costs. Clients want to know what the chances are of their pet recovering and being healthy again if they spend the money you are proposing to charge for the services you are recommending. For example, the short-term prognosis for a cat with a urinary tract blockage (often called a "plugged" or "blocked" cat) may be guarded, but if the cat makes it through anesthesia and treatment and stays on its special diet afterward, the long-term prognosis may be very good. On the other hand, the short-term prognosis for a splenectomy (spleen removal) may be very good, but if the spleen turns out to be cancerous, the long-term prognosis may be poor, and the care and money that will need to be invested after surgery may be much more than the client can emotionally or financially afford. It's impossible for clients to make informed decisions without all the facts.

Following is a list of rules to follow when estimating medical procedures for pet owners:

1. **Be honest with your clients and don't surprise them.** The client has a right to an accurate estimate, an accurate prognosis, both long- and short-term, and an accurate idea of the care needs the pet will have once it returns home.

    Estimates are to be given for both medical and surgical procedures. The rule of thumb is, if the patient enters the hospital, the owner needs an estimate. Don't forget estimates for X-rays, blood testing, and outpatient care, such as a case being treated for vomiting or diarrhea on an outpatient basis. What will it cost today? What will it cost if treatments need to be repeated tomorrow?

2. **Always estimate high.** The client will be much happier to pay less than the estimate than he or she will to pay more than the estimate. Also, you may have left something off the estimate, underestimated the time or skill the procedure would require, or discounted something you shouldn't have. For all nonroutine surgeries give a range on the consent form the client signs as well as the itemized estimate with an exact amount. Never promise that the itemized estimate will be the total on the invoice. The pet may need additional pain medication, an injection for vomiting, or

additional anesthetic and surgery time. The range on the consent form should start with the total on the estimate printout.

For example, if you put in an estimate for a cruciate repair and the total on the computer printout is $1,521.98, you would write on the consent form the owner signs that the estimate is $1,525–$2,125. Add at least 10 to 15 percent to the total for the high end of the range. The more nebulous the procedure, the wider the range will be. If applicable, create a second worst-case estimate to use as the high end of the range. An example of this would be a dental cleaning estimate and then a separate one for extracting that broken tooth if the dental radiograph shows it's abscessed.

3. **Do not compromise the level of care you are offering because you're afraid of how the owners will react to the bill.** Your job is to tell the client what the patient needs to get better as quickly as possible and with the least amount of risk and pain. How will you feel if you were afraid to offer the ECG and the pet died under anesthesia? How would you want things done if this were your own pet? Ask the client if this is the level of care he or she wants for the pet. If it is, help the client find a way to pay for it.

    You may need to offer a lower-cost option if the client honestly can't afford all of your recommendations. Explain the increased risks and/or increased care that will result from taking that route. If he or she can't afford the abscess surgery, for example, can he or she afford antibiotics and two recheck exams?

4. **If the patient will suffer greatly or die without the care you are recommending, make sure the owner understands this.** In many cases, it is better to put a pet to sleep than to forgo needed care. Do not make the owner feel guilty for not being able to afford care or not being able to do needed aftercare. Some owners have to decide between veterinary care for their pets and shoes for their children. In addition, not every owner can stomach watching a pet go through complicated or repeated medical procedures. It is the owner's right to make decisions about his or her pet even if it isn't the same decision you would make. That's life. Support the client's decision whenever you possibly can.

5. **Once a choice is made and the treatment or surgery is under way, call the client immediately if the charges exceed the estimate.** Do not let

the client discover that the bill is higher at checkout time. This puts the receptionist in an awkward situation, and other clients may overhear the owner's tirade. Ultimately, the client may decide to look for a new vet.

6. **Do not undercharge the owner to stay within an inaccurate estimate.** This can cost the clinic thousands of dollars each year. It simply should not happen. Double-check your estimate to help prevent it.

7. **Think carefully about the procedure you are giving the estimate for.** Will it be painful? Need a bandage? A drain? A biopsy? Could it lead to infection? Have you put the pain medication, bandages, drains, histopathology, and antibiotics on the estimate?

   What about follow-up care? Recheck exams and office visits, bandage changes, urine rechecks, splint repairs, pin removals, and all other follow-up charges must be estimated as well.

8. **Be sure to include ancillary services.** If you add a heartworm test and pills, that may add a large sum to the bill. Vaccines, nail trims, microchipping, stool checks, ear cleaning, and other fees must also be on the owner's estimate of services.

   While the animal is in the hospital or under anesthesia is an ideal time to do these extra procedures. Don't forget to ask if the abscessed cat can be neutered, if the pet needs a dental cleaning with that lump removal, or if the client would like the pet to get that Bordetella vaccination that is due soon.

9. **Consider what will make the anesthetic safer.** Is this pet old, or a breed prone to cardiomyopathy? How about an ECG? Is the pre-anesthetic chemistry panel enough, or should you add a CBC, a bile acids level, or a test for coagulopathy?

10. **Work out payment arrangements before starting the procedure.** Ask new clients for a down payment before any major procedures are undertaken. If you are making any payment agreements with the client, clear them with the accounts manager beforehand.

11. **Beware of any client who says, "I don't care how much it costs."** This frequently translates as "I don't intend to pay the bill anyway." Gently insist on going over the estimate anyway ("According to our clinic policy we

have to explain the estimate to you"), require a signature, and ask for a down payment of at least 50 percent of the low end of the estimate range.

12. **For serious surgeries and illnesses, provide a detailed form to help make procedures and their risks understandable.** For example, see the client form entitled "Estimate for Surgery/Anesthesia/Treatment" at the end of this section.

13. **Make sure you are clear on both a top and a bottom number.** It is human nature to hear only the best-case scenario. Clients will remember the $100 in the estimate of $100 to $150, but they will miss the $150. Again, write everything down.

14. **Remain professional but direct.** Don't cringe or hesitate when discussing money or you will appear dishonest. At checkout or when there are complications and the bill is higher than the estimate, as with estimates, it pays to be honest and straightforward. Don't beat around the bush. You can come right out and acknowledge that "Mindy had 12 infected teeth that had to be extracted. This bill is really going to be high. Are you ready for the grand total?" For optional testing or extra services, say, for example, "Last year you said you couldn't afford to do this procedure. Are your finances better this year so we can get Buffy tested for feline leukemia?"

15. **Plan your response to complaints.** If the client says, "Boy, this bill was sure high," come back with something like "Yes, we're going to have to name a parking space after you," or "We appreciate the good care you've given your pet to make him better."

    Your client's comments about price are often not complaints at all. They are just observations. Maybe the client is bragging to other clients in the waiting room about how much money he or she can afford to spend on the pet. As long as you acknowledge their comments or concerns and praise them for taking such good care of their pets, most of your clients will keep coming back.

16. **Don't let your own finances influence your recommendations to clients.** If you cringe over a $220 bill because your own checkbook contains only $189, you come across to the client as being tentative and unsure. The client starts wondering, "Did they overcharge me? Was I stupid

to have agreed to this procedure? Was that pre-anesthetic panel really necessary?"

Once you have gone over the estimate and obtained the client's signature, made payment arrangements, and, if necessary, taken a down payment, be sure you have a current telephone number for him or her. Unless you have to call the client to provide an update, the next time you deal with money matters with this client it will be time to present the invoice. A sample estimate form is provided at the end of this section and online at: <<TK website address>>.

PRESENTING INVOICES TO CLIENTS

Use effective phrases and confident body language when presenting bills to clients. Make eye contact, square your shoulders, and speak in a confident tone. You can say, for example, "Fluffy did great today and it looks like she didn't need any extractions after all. Let's see . . . the cost is $785. Would you like to take care of that with cash, check, or a credit or debit card?"

Sometimes clients want a higher level of care than they can afford—or perhaps they didn't intend to pay you in the first place. Here are some guidelines to help ensure that good care is paid for by the client and not by the clinic:

1. **Be firm.** For clients who "did not bring the checkbook" or "do not have enough cash," remind them that you accept credit cards. Keep saying over and over, "We need to get a payment today, Mr. Jones," until they come up with a plan to get you the money. Don't be afraid to repeat yourself!

    If the bill has not been paid, do not give the client items such as food or medication (unless a doctor says it's all right) until he or she returns with a payment. You can say, "We'll hold these items for you until you return."
2. **Use the 48-hour rule.** Some clients may offer to "stop back later" and pay. Consider having them sign a form that states they must pay in full within 48 hours to avoid a service charge. Put a callback reminder into your computer to check on the account when the 48 hours have passed.
3. **Get documentation according to your hospital's protocols.** To pursue a client in small claims court, your state may require that you have a client's driver's license number or Social Security number.

4. **Arrange for payment when the pet's owner is not the one who brings the pet in.** Sometimes a friend or relative brings the pet in for the procedure or visit. Ideally, you would know about this at check-in time. You could ask whether the owner sent along a check or credit card number before taking the patient to the exam room, and contact the owner at work, if necessary, to obtain one. Unless it is an emergency, you are under no obligation to provide services for a client who made no arrangements for payment. If you don't realize until checkout that the owner is not present, you can ask whoever brought the pet in to fill out and sign the payment form.

    If the person who brought the pet to you is an adult and your practice doesn't send monthly billing statements, he or she is still responsible for payment, just as he or she would be if buying groceries for you. You may have no way of verifying who the legal owner of the pet is or whose responsibility it is to pay the bill. That's their problem to resolve. You just need a payment, if your hospital's policy is payment at time of service.

    You may be in a pickle if the pet is brought in by a minor. No major procedures should be performed on a pet without an adult's consent. It is difficult to pursue a minor into collections or small claims court for an unpaid bill. Make sure any minors are aware of the cost of services and confirm that they have the money to pay for them. Try to contact a parent or guardian by phone, if necessary.

5. **Follow up on past-due accounts.** If a client's account is getting behind, it usually becomes the job of a manager to sit down with that client as soon as possible and have a frank discussion about payment for services. Do not let a client get in over his or her head. Clients lose sight of reality when they are worried about beloved pets or when they have multiple pets needing multiple things done, and they sometimes lose track of the total amount they are spending. They need to be realistic about the level of care they can afford. Again, it's not the practice's function to be a lending institution. Most animal hospitals cannot afford to have large debts outstanding. Someone will need to work out a payment plan with these clients that they can realistically meet.

6. **Don't be pulled into an argument with the client.** Given the stresses clients are often under at the veterinary clinic, it is understandable that they sometimes come across as difficult, abrasive, or short-tempered when discussing money. Your job in these situations is not to defend yourself, or even to be right. Your job is to make the client feel more at ease with the situation, explain carefully what the costs and payment policies are, and then solve the problem to keep the customer.

Sometimes, discussions about money issues are much easier than anticipated. Most clients know that you have bills to pay, too. They just need to have a clear understanding of what the rules are and what the price will be for your services. As long as your team is straightforward and the options are explained in detail to them, most people are happy to pay what they owe.

PRO BONO CARE

Occasionally your hospital may treat a patient that everyone agrees deserves more care than its owner can afford. It might be an abandoned dog with a broken leg, a cat that needs surgery owned by a little old lady on Social Security, or a sick bird who needs a new home because its owner has passed away.

> Be honest with your clients and don't surprise them.

Helping these patients get the care they need makes a hospital team feel wonderful. Start a fund for these sorts of patients and ask your clients and coworkers to contribute to it. Find a new home for the pet, if necessary, and donate care. You might be able to work out a deal with the local animal shelter to rehome the pet once you've treated it. Work with the American Animal Hospital Association's Helping Pets Fund, which provides money to accredited hospitals and their clients for major medical expenses (up to one patient per hospital per year). Do whatever works for those deserving patients, because bending over backward to help an animal that desperately needs it is very rewarding for a clinic team. That feeling is what inspired most of us to enter the field of animal care in the first place. Sometimes you need to recapture the feeling that you are helping to relieve suffering and promoting the bond between people and animals.

RESOURCES

American Animal Hospital Association. "AAHA Seal of Acceptance," www.aahanet.org/eweb/dynamicpage.aspx?site=resources&webcode=SealofAcceptance. The AAHA Seal of Acceptance means that a "pet health insurance company's high-deductible policies meet AAHA recommendations."

CareCredit, www.CareCredit.com. CareCredit provides credit cards for use at veterinary hospitals as well as for human dental- and eye-care services. They offer interest-free payment plans that can help clients to afford procedures they would not be able to pay for all at once.

DVM360, www.dvm360.com. This site has articles on money management topics. Under the "Business Center" menu, click on "Client Handouts" and look for "Final Collection Letter," "Payment Agreement Form," "Compare Pet Insurance Plans," "Top 4 Reasons Pet Insurance Claims Are Denied," and a "Compassionate Care Fund" protocol and application. Under "Practice Operations Forms," you'll find "Smooth Out Pet Insurance Wrinkles with These Protocols" and "Payment and Billing Policy."

Pet Insurance Review, www.PetInsuranceReview.com. This site has a chart of currently available pet insurance companies and plans so that clients can compare policies.

Robertson, Stacey. 2002. "Collecting Payment." *Veterinary Economics*, October 1.

Rothstein, Jeff. 2006. "Coping with Credit Cards." *Veterinary Economics*, November 1.

Volk, John, and Christine Merle. 2009. "A Veterinarian's Guide to Pet Health Insurance." National Commission on Veterinary Economic Issues, www.ncvei.org/article.aspx?id=41.

"When Clients Can't Pay." 2009. *Veterinary Economics*, August 1.

ESTIMATE FOR SURGERY/ANESTHESIA/TREATMENT

All anesthetic procedures and surgeries entail risk. Occasionally, patients can experience adverse effects from virtually any procedure. However, the risks of problems from anesthesia are generally much lower than the risks of untreated diseases or problems.

The procedure recommended for your pet is ....

This entails ....

....

....

Ancillary/supportive/additional items necessary along with the procedure are:

- ☐ Intravenous fluids via catheter
- ☐ Subcutaneous fluids
- ☐ Blood testing
- ☐ Urine testing
- ☐ Pathology samples sent to a laboratory
- ☐ Bandages
- ☐ Cast/splint
- ☐ Urinary catheter
- ☐ Intensive hospital care
- ☐ Special diet
- ☐ Medications sent home
- ☐ Pain medications
- ☐ Other medications
- ☐ Elizabethan collar/harness to prevent chewing
- ☐ Drains to remove pus or other fluids
- ☐ Isolation/special cleaning procedures
- ☐ Recheck X-rays
- ☐ Other ....

Risk assessments help to give us an idea of the likelihood of problems from a procedure. We rate risks on a scale of I to V.

Class I risk is the lowest. For Class I procedures, the animal is believed to be young and healthy and the surgery is considered to be elective. Spays, neuters, declaws, and dentistries on young pets are usually Class I.

In **Class II**, the pet is believed to be healthy but the procedure is not elective. Repairing a broken leg on a young dog would be a Class II procedure.

In **Class III**, there are health problems with the pet that make the procedure more risky, but the patient has no obvious signs of illness. Advanced age, heart or kidney disease, epilepsy, and infection are examples of problems that increase the patient's risk to Class III. Dentistries in elderly pets and treating cat bite abscesses are Class III procedures. Any pet for which we do not have pre-anesthetic blood test results is automatically a Class III category or higher.

Class IV patients have overt signs of disease. Surgery or medical care is needed to treat a disease or problem, but the disease itself has made the animal ill and the procedure or outcome is somewhat risky. Class IV procedures include exploratory surgeries, cancer surgery, surgery to treat severe infections, catheterization to relieve a urinary obstruction, IV fluid therapy for gastrointestinal illness, and many others.

In **Class V**, the pet is gravely ill and needs a procedure or treatment to save its life. The prognosis may be guarded to poor. Without the procedure the pet will very likely die, but the necessary procedure is very risky also, or the treatment may not be successful.

Your pet's procedure is graded ....

The short-term prognosis is ....

The long-term prognosis, assuming the procedure is successful, is ....

....

The cost of any procedure will vary depending on the health of the pet and the response to treatment. Some animals need more fluids or pain medication than others. Laboratory testing, length of anesthetic and surgery time, and any complications encountered will affect the total price. Medications and food needed upon discharge and length of stay in the hospital also may vary. Emergencies and after-hours surgeries increase costs.

Our estimate for (pet's name)...

for this procedure, scheduled/given on (date) .... is between $..................... and $.....................

We will do our best to keep you informed of accumulating charges and any change in the original estimate if problems develop.

☐ I will need to arrange a payment plan to pay for this procedure. (All payment agreements are subject to credit approval by the hospital.)

☐ I accept the above estimate and authorize you to perform the listed procedure(s).

....
SIGNATURE

☐ I refuse the above recommended procedure.
  (If other alternatives exist, the doctor will go over these with you.)

....
SIGNATURE

PAYMENT AGREEMENT

Today's Date ....

☐ I agree to pay the .... Animal Hospital $ ....
for services and/or supplies (medication, food, etc.) given to my pet(s). I understand that a $25 service charge will be added if I do not pay within 48 hours.

☐ I understand that as a responsible adult who has requested veterinary services for a pet, I am, under law, liable for payment of $ .... for those services, regardless of who the actual owner of the pet is. Therefore, I also understand that if payment for these services is not received from the owner, ... Animal Hospital will pursue me for payment. A $25 service charge will be added if payment is not received within 48 hours.

....
NAME (PLEASE PRINT)

....
HOME PHONE NUMBER

....
DRIVER'S LICENSE NUMBER

....
SOCIAL SECURITY NUMBER

....
DATE OF BIRTH

....
SIGNATURE

OFFICE USE ONLY:

employee initials ....

callback entered ....

NUTRITION AND NUTRACEUTICALS

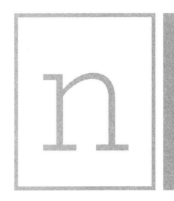

One of the most common questions clients will ask you is "What should I feed my pet?" And it's a great question, because it deals with the most important contribution a client makes to a pet's health and well-being on a daily basis: diet. It's important to be ready with a good answer.

With pet foods, as with many other things, consumers may find more long-term value in specialty pet food brands. Clients should understand that some inexpensive dog and cat foods contain low-quality ingredients. They are not well digested and may have deficiencies or excesses in vital nutrients. Scientists working in research laboratory settings have found that many generic and store-brand foods do not actually contain the level of nutrition stated on their labels.

Unfortunately, some premium pet-store foods are not always what they claim to be. Long ingredient lists name a number of ingredients—including chicory, probiotics, fruits and vegetables, licorice, and kelp—that are supposed to improve health, but the claims aren't always backed up by scientific studies. Many smaller brands may be produced in manufacturing plants that produce many different brands, so crossover contamination from one line of food to another, ingredient substitutions may be common.

If a pet-food company doesn't conduct research on its foods or have strict quality control, its executives may not know that its calcium source is contaminated with lead or that those chicken by-products are all beaks and feet. When deciding what to recommend, choose reputable companies that do their research well, and beware of unsupported claims.

Probiotics, for example, are so-called good bacteria, the kind that live in our intestines and help us to digest our food. When added to pet food or as supplements, they are meant to survive passage through the stomach into the gastrointestinal tract, where they would be expected to multiply and produce positive effects. They are considered food supplements and are not regulated by any government agency. A study that analyzed 19 brands of pet food that claimed to contain probiotics found that most of them did not contain the bacterial species listed on the label and none contained an amount sufficient to be useful. Unfortunately, pet owners often waste their money purchasing products that are worthless. It's our job to help them choose diets and supplements that actually are helpful (Gorbach 2000; Weese and Arroyo 2003).

To help them get the nutrition they are paying for, tell clients to choose a well-known name brand, preferably one that has its own laboratories and publishes nutritional studies. The best foods are tested extensively to meet rigid standards with no ingredient substitutions. They contain controlled levels of key nutrients such as fat, protein, phosphorus, and magnesium to help reduce the risk of obesity and urinary tract disease. Many diseases are caused by excesses of nutrients like these—nutritional deficiencies are not nearly as common as problems from too much food or too much of a certain ingredient. The products should also be produced in the company's own plants.

The pet will do best if the client chooses a complete food appropriate for the pet's age and activity level and sticks with it. For a puppy or kitten, this means puppy or kitten food. For a large-breed puppy it's a large-breed puppy formula. For older pets, "senior" food is usually best. Changing a pet's diet won't produce immediate results. It usually takes about six weeks to see a change in a pet's skin or coat after a diet change.

Be wary of label claims for senior or "lite" diets, however. Dry dog foods labeled "light," "lite," "low calorie," or "less calorie" have calorie counts varying from 217 to 440 calories per cup, and the recommended intake printed on the bag can vary from 0.73 to 1.47 times the dog's resting energy requirements (Freeman and Linder 2010). In other words, one cup of one brand could have twice as many calories as one cup of another; if an owner feeds the pet an amount according to the label, it may not always be the correct amount for the pet. Studies on various aspects of pet foods, including probiotic content, ingredients present compared with ingredients listed on the label, and compliance with federal guidelines for caloric content, have all shown major discrepancies. It's hard to believe that a food can have chicken listed as the first ingredient yet have no poultry DNA in it whatsoever, but it has happened (Jonker et al. 2008; Fujimura et al. 2008).

Warn clients that feeding their pets too many treats is as bad for them as it is for us. Feeding a pet more treats means feeding it less of the regular, well-balanced food it should be eating. Treats should never make up more than 10 percent of the daily food intake. Many treats are also loaded with salt, artificial colorings, and flavorings that pets don't need. If clients want to feed their pets treats, recommend healthy ones. Many dogs like carrots, for example, and for cats a small bit of tuna or chicken may be a good treat if their kidneys are healthy.

A cup or scoop of food may be much larger or smaller in a client's mind than in yours, so be sure clients are accurately measuring the amount they are feeding their pets with an actual measuring cup. Provide a plastic measuring cup for this purpose, if possible. Also, if a canned equivalent is available and the owner likes to mix dry food with wet food, be sure to let the owners know this, so they don't undercut the special diet by adding nontherapeutic food to it.

It can be difficult to switch a pet from one food to another. If you recommend a food change to clients, be sure to tell them to mix the old food in with

FOODS THAT ARE TOXIC TO PETS

Some human foods are toxic to pets, including chocolate, grapes and raisins, macadamia nuts, onions, rising bread dough, and any product containing the artificial sweetener Xylitol. Clients should also avoid giving their pets human foods that are high in fat or salt.

the new for a time instead of abruptly switching from one to another. This strategy helps to prevent diarrhea and makes the switch less noticeable to the pet. In cats, especially, slower transitions are usually more effective than sudden changes.

Research shows that cats are very attuned to the shape and texture of a food—more so than to its flavor (Hand et al. 2010). Cats become accustomed to the way a particular shape and size of nugget feels in their mouths and are reluctant to change foods. Warn owners of this reason for "finicky" behavior ahead of time—their cats will probably need some time to grow accustomed to the new food. Both cat and dog owners can mix some canned food in with the dry if the pet isn't too excited about its new diet.

It's a good idea for pet owners to switch foods at least a few times when a pet is young so that it learns to eat more than one size and shape of nugget and will be less reluctant to change foods later on. Give owners several good options so they can go back and forth a time or two.

Your clinic probably recommends or sells specific brands that the veterinarian feels are nutritionally superior to grocery-store brands. Be enthusiastic about these foods when recommending them, because good nutrition is a major factor in the health of the pets you see. Read up on the diets you sell and talk with the company's sales representatives so you can be knowledgeable about the products you promote. Many companies provide videos and nutritional education kits so you can learn more about basic pet nutrition. Be sure you take advantage of these resources.

It's easy to be enthusiastic about the wonderful therapeutic diets available now. We can prevent and cure many diseases and prolong a pet's life expectancy simply by managing its diet. Kidney, liver, and heart disease; feline urinary tract problems; cancer; food allergies; dry skin; obesity; colitis; constipation; vomiting and diarrhea; dental tartar; and weight loss are just some of the problems addressed by nutritional support. Millions of pets are alive and well today solely because they are eating the right foods. One doctor from Nestlé Purina PetCare was quoted in *Veterinary Practice News* as saying, "One way to approach the cost of feeding a therapeutic diet is to consider that the benefits of the diet and improved pet health may mean fewer veterinary visits and bills for the related medical issue. Purina's HA Canine Formula for pets is a costly diet, but it works. A successful therapeutic diet means a healthier pet" (Tremayne 2010).

> One doctor from Nestlé Purina PetCare said, "One way to approach the cost of feeding a therapeutic diet is to consider that the benefits of the diet and improved pet health may mean fewer veterinary visits and bills for the related medical issue."

When a client is advised that a diet change is necessary, be sure they understand why. They need to know what treats or snacks are still safe for the pet, how much of the new food to give the pet, and how fast to switch from one food to the other. They also need to know whether a recheck is needed, and if so, when and why. The veterinarian may need to reweigh the pet to see how it is doing on its new diet, or repeat blood or urine tests. As always, these things should be written down. The client should be given written instructions to follow at home to refer to when feeding the pet. It's important for clients to be able to refer to these while establishing the new routine.

Be enthusiastic and creative.

Many owners undercut their nutritional efforts by feeding their pets prescription dry foods but adding grocery-store canned foods or table food to it. Explain to clients why this is counterproductive. Even a small amount of a regular food can reduce or negate the positive effects of the therapeutic diet. For example, if the pet needs a low-sodium diet for heart disease but the pet owner gives the dog salty snacks as treats, he or she is adding all the sodium back into the diet that the therapeutic diet eliminated. Similarly, it doesn't take much of an 80 percent–protein canned cat food from the grocery store to put the cat with kidney disease over its protein limit of 24 percent.

You might want to make up a chart that lists all the foods you sell and what each diet is designed to accomplish or counter. You can also list what the alternatives are if the pet doesn't like the food and which foods are available in canned form, dry form, or both. A sample food-chart entry, this one for Hill's K/D food, is shown below.

FOOD CHART

Diet	Use	Canned/Dry	Alternatives
K/D	Kidney or liver disease	Both	CNM-NF, Iams Veterinary, Formula Renal Early Stage, Royal Canin

NUTRACEUTICALS

Along with basic nutritional knowledge, you must also have a working knowledge of nutritional supplements, called *nutraceuticals* in the veterinary field. Nutraceuticals are defined by the North American Veterinary Neutraceutical Council as "[nondrug] substances produced in a purified or extracted form and administered orally." Nutraceuticals provide chemicals required for normal body structure and function, with the intent of improving health and well-being. These include SaME, MSM, glucosamine, fatty acids, prebiotics, probiotics, and antioxidants, among other things. Sometimes, as with Hill's J/D, the nutraceutical is contained in the food. Other supplements, such as glucosamine, would usually be sold separately.

About 50 percent of Americans regularly use supplements, and about 10 percent of pets are taking them, too. An estimated 65 percent of pet owners whose pets have cancer are giving them supplements, usually without the knowledge of the veterinarian (Freeman et al. 2006; Lana et al. 2006). Nutraceuticals have characteristics of both nutrients and pharmaceuticals, though they are not regulated as either of these. The companies that make them cannot claim that they treat or cure disease—if they did, the U.S. Food and Drug Administration (FDA) would insist on classifying them as drugs and require them to go through a rigorous testing and approval process. Instead, they are used as "complementary management options" that "promote improved body function and assist in long-term management of certain chronic conditions." This vague verbiage allows them to fly under the radar of the drug regulatory system.

Safety, efficacy, and manufacturing standards are not well regulated for nutraceuticals. Product labeling is an issue because these products often do not contain the labeled ingredients in the stated amounts. In other words, as with pet foods, what it says on the label may not be what is in the bottle. Other ingredients may be present that aren't listed on the label at all. Most of these products won't hurt pets, but they may not be helping them either. In a study of over-the-counter glucosamine supplements for humans, only two of 60 brands tested actually contained the same ingredients in the same amounts as listed on the label (ConsumerLab.com 2009a, 2009b).

Nutraceutical manufacturers are not required to report "adverse events" in patients taking these products. Manufacturing standards and quality control are thus up to the individual manufacturer. As we have discovered during pet-food recalls in recent years, we don't always know where ingredients in unregulated products really come from. Many of these products or the ingredients used in them come from overseas, where regulations and quality-control standards are not always as high as in the United States.

The most common nutraceuticals used in veterinary medicine are glucosamine and chondroitin sulfate. Both are found in many, many brands of supplements and may be listed on dog-food labels as well. Glucosamine is a normal ingredient that has always been present in pet food because it is found in the meat by-products used in pet foods. The small amounts present naturally are not enough to provide a therapeutic benefit, however. If a pet-food label says "contains glucosamine," that in itself does not mean the pet is getting the amount it needs from that food. The form of glucosamine is important as well. The hydrochloride (HCl) form is more readily absorbed by dogs than the sulfate form, but you may not be able to tell by the pet-food label which type is present.

Over-the-counter pet foods do not have these ingredients in sufficient amounts to be considered therapeutic. In fact, having them in these amounts would be illegal because then the diet would be classified as a drug as well as a food and could no longer be sold over the counter. In other words, only prescription diets that are regulated can have therapeutic amounts of medical-use ingredients.

NUTRIGENOMICS: A NEW NUTRITIONAL SCIENCE

Some of the most interesting research being done in the field of nutrition today is on how various nutrients affect the functioning of individual cells. Every cell in our bodies contains the same DNA, and all the instructions for producing the different structures and processes the body uses and performs are contained in that genetic code. Each cell, however, only expresses part of the DNA.

Many drugs affect gene expression. Aspirin, for example, decreases the cells' manufacture of prostaglandins, proteins that cause pain and inflammation. Nutrients can do this, too. Omega-3 fatty acids turn off the genes expressing inflammation and turn on ones that produce anti-inflammatory genes instead. When you feed a pet a fatty acid–rich diet or add a supplement containing fatty acids, it takes many weeks to see the effect. Once that happens, though, the cells will function differently, producing more anti-inflammatory chemicals and fewer inflammatory ones. As this happens, symptoms of inflammation, such as arthritis pain, itchy skin, and poor brain function, should improve.

As scientists unravel the mysteries of how these effects occur inside the cell, they are opening up a fascinating new way for us to tackle various disease problems. Research is under way to formulate diets that program cells to burn fat instead of store it, to decrease inflammation in the pancreas, or to reduce intestinal inflammation and diarrhea in animals with inflammatory bowel disease. In the years to come, instead of giving our pets drugs to treat diseases, we may be feeding them special diets formulated to turn genes on or off inside cells in order to improve the health and function of the body.

The field of nutrition is a dynamic and interesting one. New discoveries about essential nutrients and vitamins continue to be made, and new diets that use these discoveries appear on a regular basis. Sometimes it can be difficult to keep up with all of them. Try to stay organized and informed so you can phase in these new products and recommendations and convey new nutritional advances to clients with pets that need them.

RESOURCES

American Animal Hospital Association. "AAHA Nutritional Assessment Guidelines for Dogs and Cats." www.aahanet.org/resources/NutritionalGuidelines.aspx.

American College of Veterinary Nutrition, www.acvn.org.

DVM360, www.dvm360.com. Here you can find a nutrition questionnaire and a nutritional supplement handout. Look in "Client Handouts" under the "Business Center" menu.

DVM Consulting, Balance IT website, www.balanceit.com. This website has a database on thousands of pet foods, software to compare and contrast them, and a method of creating custom feeding plans and weight-loss programs. DVM Consulting offers a subscription service called "Autobalancer" that is designed to help pet owners and vets balance animal diets for nutrient content. It also incorporates supplements. There are two areas of the website, one for pet owners and the other for veterinarians.

Hand, Michael S., Craig D. Thatcher, Rebecca L. Remillard, Phillip Roundebush, and Bruce J. Novotny. 2010. *Small Animal Clinical Nutrition*, 5th ed. Topeka, KS: Mark Morris Institute.

Kirk, Claudia A., ed. 2006. "Dietary Management and Nutrition." *Veterinary Clinics of North America: Small Animal Practice* 36, no. 6 (November), special issue. See http://vetsmall.theclinics.com/issues/contents?issue_key=S0195-5616%2806%29X0029-3.

National Research Council (NRC), www.nal.usda.gov/fnic/foodcomp/search/. The NRC publishes guides on the nutrient needs of animals.

"Plentiful Food Sales." 2008. *Veterinary Economics*, March 1.

University of California at Davis Veterinary Medicine, www.vmth.ucdavis.edu. UC Davis's veterinary school offers lots of handouts. Topics include nutritional management of chronic kidney disease, gastrointestinal disease, urolithiasis, diabetes, hepatitis, and weight control.

OVER-THE-COUNTER SALES

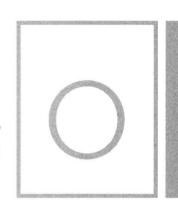

Your clients trust you to know about animal care and to recommend the best products for their pets. When your client asks you which shampoo would be best for Flopsey, he or she doesn't want to hear you say, "Oh, any of those would be fine," or "I really don't know." Often clients trust a lay team member more than they trust the veterinarian on over-the-counter (OTC) items. The entire team needs to live up to that trust and give honest, truthful recommendations.

Your clients want to know what you use on your own pets. If you wouldn't use it on your own pet, why would you sell it to a client? Be honest with your clients. Tell them which products you use with your own pet and why. The most successful veterinary OTC salespeople know the products they sell and can tell customers all about them: "This shampoo really smells great but this one gets a white coat whiter," or "These are the kind of nail clippers that work best on large dogs," or "My dog's coat is so much nicer since I started her on this fatty acid supplement. I know it will work great for you, too."

If clients don't need a product, tell them so. They will trust you more the next time, when you think they do need something. Conversely, if you have a product you know would benefit their pet, don't be shy about telling clients so. Even if they don't buy it this time, they still may appreciate the information and buy it the next time.

Be honest with your clients. Tell them which products you use with your own pet and why.

If you are new to veterinary medicine, you may not know a lot about the products on your shelves. You will need to read labels, try things on your own animals, and watch what other team members are selling. Ask lots of questions. You might want to start a file or notebook on the products you sell and put flyers and other product information inside to reference when you need it. Make a list of the items you don't know much about, one shelf or item at a time, and check them off as you learn about them. Or make up index cards on each product or a cheat sheet.

OTC sales are a great place to use a communication tool I call a "value statement." Value statements help us to communicate to our clients the value of our products or services both to them and to their pets. They increase the perception of our value and also add to clients' perception that we care. Value statements can be about what our values are as a practice (what we believe is good care) as well as about what goes into a service or product that makes it costly and why it's worth the money. They can be used on the phone or in person.

An example of a value statement for a service would be this script that a client relations specialist might use when clients call to ask the price of a spay procedure: "We use isofluorane, the safest gas anesthesia, because we feel it's very important to ensure our patients' safety. We use a clean, sterile surgery pack for every patient, and we have certified technicians administering the anesthesia. These steps will help make sure that Princess will be safe and comfortable during this procedure."

To make a product value statement, you need to know a bit about the product, how it is used, and why your hospital recommends it. "This flea preventive works great and it's very safe, which is why we recommend it over store brands. Because it's waterproof it won't wash off, so it's perfect for dogs, like your Rocky, who swim. Let me show you how to apply it."

Here are some rules for value statements:

1. **Always precede a price with a value statement.** For example, "This product costs more than what you would find at the store but it's safer and more effective. We have a buy six, get one free offer right now, which would last you the rest of the season. The price per tube is $_____, or with six plus one free it would be $_____."
2. **If a client questions the cost of an item, always give a value statement.** "You know, I used to think J/D was expensive, too, until my dog developed arthritis and I found out how much better he felt once he was eating it. Did you know that most dogs eating J/D need less of their expensive prescription medication?"
3. **If a client seems hesitant or unsure about something, always give a value statement.** When a client seems hesitant, you can acknowledge his or her feelings when you make the value statement and offer to answer questions. For example, you might say, "Dr. Smith thinks this is the best product for Rocky and it works great for my dog, too. Do you have any questions about it?" or "You seem to be hesitating. Could I explain something better for you?"
4. **If you are offering something new to the client, always give a value statement.** You can also repeat your explanation of what the item is. "I see that you haven't used Frontline before. It works really well and it's very safe. Let me show you how to put it on."
5. **Always try to add a caring or empathetic statement to your explanation.** "I know you are worried about Molly's itchy skin. She seems very uncomfortable. This shampoo should really help."
6. **Differentiate yourself from other clinics.** "We only stock products that we feel comfortable using on our own pets." "Most clinics don't carry the number of behavior products that we do. There are some really neat puzzle toys available now for enrichment and training."
7. **Always ask if the client has questions or concerns.** The whole purpose of the value statement is to make sure the client understands what he or she will be paying for. Never rush your explanation, and be sure you have covered as much as the client seems to want to know. Be sensitive to the client's body language and questions and don't push someone to buy anything he or she doesn't really want or need.

Value statements provide repetition of and reinforcement for the doctor's recommendations. Working together, each person on the veterinary team supports the goals of the practice and reinforces the messages sent to clients.

A fun exercise to do at a team meeting is to have each person choose an OTC item that he or she uses or knows about and give a value statement for it to the rest of the group. Many times products have benefits or uses that some team members are aware of but others are not.

Don't wait for someone to hold your hand and tell you what to sell and how to sell it. Unfortunately, veterinarians, technicians, and many practice managers have no training in sales or marketing, so your coworkers may not be able to teach you what you need to know. You may need to be proactive about educating yourself. Most sales representatives will give your team presentations or brochures about their products. Companies often have dinner meetings or provide lunch and a lecture at your own clinic to educate both veterinarians and team members about their products. Ask your employer about implementing a bonus plan to reward OTC sales. Remember, your clients won't buy products from you if they don't know what's available. The ultimate goal, of course, is to get more patients on better diets for improved health and to encourage clients to try products that will enhance their pets' lives. Try asking clients why they like products they are already using, too. You can learn things from them that you can later repeat to other clients.

> **Repetition is key.**

Your clients won't buy products from you if they don't know what's available.

Product displays should be neat, well organized, and dusted regularly. Clients don't like to buy the last item on a shelf, so keep the items well stocked. Bottles and other containers should come right to the front edge of the shelf, not be crowded or pushed to the back. Keep similar items near each other so clients can compare them. Be sure the shelves are well lit.

You can set up seasonal displays to highlight appropriate products and put up cards or signs notifying clients of specials or discounted items. It is important to change your displays around regularly to make them look fresh. You can also mention particular products in a newsletter. All these suggestions are part of a good retail sales program and will help you to market items to your customers.

Customers want to pick up items and hold them in their hands, and they like prices marked on the item so they don't have to ask. It's best to keep items within reach, with the most important ones at eye level.

A nice no-pressure sales technique is to discuss an item with the client in the exam room and then leave it on the table in front of him or her when you leave the room. The client can pick it up and read the label or get the price, or even take the cap off and smell it if it is a product such as a shampoo. If the client decides to purchase the item, he or she can take it up to the counter. If not, he or she can leave it there.

If clients don't get the service they want from you, they can (and probably will) go down the road to the pet store and get the same items there. The difference between you and the pet store is that your clinic hires and trains people who have a lot of knowledge about pet care. Chances are good the pet store has poorly trained, inexperienced help. You are in a position to help your clients out a great deal by steering them toward the products that will work best for them and their pets. Don't let them down!

RESOURCES

Heinke, Marsha L., and John B. McCarthy. 2001. *Practice Made Perfect: A Guide to Veterinary Practice Management*. Lakewood, CO: AAHA Press. See Chapter 12, "Marketing Your Veterinary Practice."

"Make Product Sales a Profitable Piece of Your Practice." 2008. *Veterinary Economics*, October 15.

Stowe, James D. 2004. *The Effective Veterinary Practice: Beyond Management*. Lowell Ackerman, ed. Guelph, Ontario: Lifelearn. See Chapter 8, "Professional Marketing—Retailing."

PHARMACY

Proper use of medications is very important to the health of veterinary clinic patients. If the pet owner does not store and give a medication properly, it may not be effective. Clients also need to know what side effects to watch for, when to stop giving the medication, and what to do if it doesn't seem to be working as it should. Although it is the doctor's responsibility to prescribe the medications, other members of the team will explain the doctor's instructions, provide further information and handouts, check to see if clients have questions, and emphasize the importance of administering the medication correctly. Team members may also need to demonstrate how to administer the medication to the pet, and they should be familiar with the tools that may be needed for this, such as pill poppers or Pill Pockets™.

Clients should understand why their pets need the medications prescribed. If a medication is prescribed to treat an illness, the owner should always get a handout, brochure, or copy of an article or textbook page that describes the illness, the medication, and the possible side effects of the medication. This is especially important for serious or chronic diseases. The client should also be involved in the decision-making process. An educated client is far more likely to give the medication on time and to return for recheck examinations.

Half of all human patients take the wrong medications, or take the right ones in the wrong doses, at the wrong times, or in the wrong ways, according to the Institute for Safe Medication Practices (ISMP). These inadvertent errors lead to an estimated 125,000 deaths and more than $8.5 billion in hospital costs annually in the United States. In addition, 67 percent of Americans cannot remember the names of their own medications. In order to minimize problems with medications for pets, we need to be very aware of the fact that clients are easily confused when it comes to drugs and dosages (Committee on Health Literacy 2004).

Team members should discuss prescriptions with clients when dispensing the medications and give clients written information about them at the same time. In fact, every time you dispense a drug, you can give the client a medication information sheet (MIS) like the one that appears at the end of this section. You can fill these out in advance for the different medications and simply take one out of a binder or file drawer when needed, or you can have them print out automatically when a drug is entered into the invoice. (This is not necessary for refills unless it's been a long time since the client has used a particular medication for the pet.) Digital versions of the information sheets for more than 100 common medications are also available in my *Client Education Notebook: Customized Client Education Materials to Use in Your Own Practice* (see Resources).

Whether you have a paperless system or not, however, keeping accurate and timely patient records is essential, and all team members should know how to use and update them properly. Each time a drug is refilled for a client, it must be recorded. Exam dates should also be recorded, and prescriptions should not be automatically refilled if follow-up visits have been missed. Consult the veterinarian in cases like this.

Medication information sheets not only educate clients but also protect the practice from lawsuits and decrease the number of phone calls you receive about medication side effects. Moreover, when people have their own prescriptions filled at regular pharmacies, they often get a computer printout about their medication. They expect this for their pets as well. A benefit of having these sheets is that anyone in the practice can go over the medications and possible side effects with the client—it doesn't have to be done by the doctor. Even your newest team members, using the forms, can likely explain what to

WHAT TO DO WITH OLD MEDICATIONS

Pet medications, like human medications, must be disposed of when they are no longer needed. Left sitting around, they are a hazard to children in the home and others who might mistake them for something else and accidentally take them. But they should not simply be flushed down the toilet or poured down the drain, as this pollutes our waterways and is harmful for fish and other wildlife. You can take some simple measures to help your clients dispose of them properly:

- Create a bring-back program for your hospital, so that clients can bring unused medications back to you. You can credit clients for anything in tamper-proof packaging that is still in date, such as heartworm pills still in the foil wrapper. By law, you cannot resell medications in open containers, such as a vial of pills, but sometimes the leftovers can be reusable by someone else, such as the Humane Society. You can also dispose of the leftovers properly, helping to keep hazardous or potentially abusable drugs from causing harm.
- Tell clients about pharmacies or hazardous waste collection sites in the community that have drug take-back programs.
- Instruct clients not to flush unused drugs down the drain unless the label specifically says that it is okay to do so. Instead, they can mix liquid medications with cat litter, coffee grounds, or sawdust, place the mix in a plastic bag, and dispose of it in the trash. The same thing can be done with tablet or capsule medications by crushing them and mixing them with water. This keeps the drugs from filtering into the groundwater once they are in the landfill.

If a pet has a problem that might recur, you can advise clients as to what medications they might want to keep on hand for emergencies. Having a few doses of pain medication or a partial tube of ointment sometimes comes in handy for minor problems that occur in the pet at night or on a weekend.

Some medications shouldn't be left over in the first place. Following a surgery, every dose of a pain medication should be administered even if the pet does not seem to be in pain, since it may be hard to tell when a pet is suffering and when it is not. When a course of antibiotics is cut short, recurrent infection can result. You can help to clarify these issues for clients.

watch for, whether to give the medication with or without food, and whether a cat might eat it crushed in food.

All medications carry the risk of side effects. Clients frequently have concerns or questions about a medication, especially if they have been reading about it on the Internet. It's our job to carefully explain the risks and to put them into perspective. Most common side effects are mild and temporary.

Follow-up visits may be necessary for patients on long-term medications. Especially with medications prescribed for long-term use to treat chronic diseases, such as arthritis or heart disease, there are specific problems we should be monitoring for. Some drugs can cause kidney and liver disorders, for example, so we must monitor kidney and liver function when pets take them. Estrogen-based drugs, used for female dogs with urinary incontinence, can affect the bone marrow, so a complete blood count (CBC) should be done at least once a year to make sure the marrow is still manufacturing blood cells as it should. Another incontinence drug, phenylpropanolamine, can lead to high blood pressure, so we would check the pet's blood pressure regularly. These extra precautions help to keep our patients safe while we are treating them with medication. As a member of the practice team, you will need to explain the reasons for the follow-up visits and testing to clients so that they will be more likely to keep their appointments and be involved in the care of their pets.

> **The entire team must be great communicators!**

Remember, no matter how experienced you are, mistakes happen. Always double-check the bottle and label for any medication you draw up or count out. For example, all dewormers readied by a client relations specialist or assistant in my hospital must be double-checked by another team member to

---

SAFETY WARNING

Be sure to tell clients not to substitute medications intended for humans for their pets, and vice versa. Pets have different tolerances than humans, and drug dosages also may be different between species. Such substitutions can be very dangerous.

> **KEEPING ACCURATE INVENTORY IS A GOVERNMENT REQUIREMENT**
>
> Clinics are required by law to perform a complete drug inventory at least once every two years. When clients question your hospital's dispensing fees, you can point this out: "It's very expensive to stock and maintain our drug inventory, and the government has regulations we must follow that also increase our costs." For further information on pharmacy inventory management, see the Resources listed at the end of this section.

avoid errors and catch mistakes. In addition, it is illegal to dispense a medication without a proper label. The label must contain the hospital name and phone number, the patient's name, the name and strength of the drug, and the amount and frequency of administration.

Remember, no matter how experienced you are, mistakes happen. Always double-check the bottle and label for any medication you draw up or count out.

Make sure your clients understand how often a drug should be given. If the instructions say, "Give two tablets daily," that means give them both at once, not one in the morning and one in the evening. If they say "twice daily," that means approximately 12 hours apart, not one at 8 a.m. and one at noon. If they say to use it in the ears, that doesn't mean to use it in the eyes. Clients can be remarkably scatterbrained about these things, and if they make a mistake, it could be terrible for the pet. Pharmacists' horror stories are common about patients swallowing suppositories, under- or overdosing themselves, or combining drugs that are harmful.

Some of your clients cannot read, may read poorly, or have bad eyesight. Many can read but don't bother to read the written information you give them. It is wise to ask your clients to read the drug dosage information back to you from the label of any medication to ensure they get it right. If multiple drugs are needed, write instructions on paper or give the client a daily timetable of when to give each medication. For instance, for a cat with two diseases being treated with three medications, you could write, "Give [Drug 1] and [Drug 2] at 7 a.m. At 4 p.m., give [Drug 2] again. At 7 p.m., give [Drug 1] again. At bedtime, give the last dose of [Drug 2] and one tablet of [Drug 3]." For each drug that you mention, fill in the name as it appears on the label so there can be no confusion.

> Remember, different people learn best in different ways.

Demonstrate how to apply eye or ear ointment or how to give a pill, and then have the client repeat it for you. Some of your clients have had many pets, have given many medications, and are quite good at it. Others are new at it and can learn, while others will be squeamish and unable to give the medication at all. Sometimes it's possible to use the trick of hiding pills in bits of canned cat food and then freezing them. The frozen bit of food with the pill inside can slide down a pet's throat easily without leaving the bitter taste of medicine behind. Another trick is to put several medications in a single gel cap so they can all be administered at once.

Admittedly, it can be difficult to give a dog or cat its medication, especially when the pet was not trained to let the owner handle its mouth when it was a

---

WARNING ON INTERNET PHARMACIES

Counterfeit and mislabeled medications are commonly sold over the Internet. To educate your clients about why they should purchase prescription products directly from their veterinarian, the U.S. Food and Drug Administration, the National Association of Boards of Pharmacy, and the American Veterinary Medical Association have put together a brochure for clients entitled "Online Pet Pharmacies. Protect Yourself and Your Pet: Be A.W.A.R.E." You can download it at www.fda.gov/AnimalVeterinary/ ResourcesforYou/animalhealthliteracy/ucm203000.htm. Visit any of these websites for more information: www.fda.gov/Drugs.htm, www.nabp.net, and www.avma.org/ issues/prescribing/default.asp.

puppy or kitten. Obedience training and socialization for young pets can help set the stage for taking medications. As it is, many people are afraid to push a pill down a pet's throat—or are even afraid of the pet, period. What a wonderful world it would be if patients took their medicine willingly!

In serious cases, you can offer to let the client bring the pet in every day for its medicine, or the animal could be boarded for a few days, if necessary. Show the client how to wrap a cat with a towel into a "kitty burrito" for easy administration of eye medication or eardrops. Order a muzzle for these pets, or sell the client a "pill popper." For some pets, it is easier to give an injection than to give pills. You can also offer to crush tablets into liquid or order a suspension of the medication from a compounding pharmacy. Ask if a friend or neighbor can help the client. Do whatever you need to do to make giving the medication possible for the client—otherwise, the patient simply won't get the care it needs.

Clients spend a lot of money at your clinic on medications. In fact, it's probably one of the biggest profit centers in your practice. Make sure the pets actually receive the medications the owners are paying for.

RESOURCES

American Veterinary Medical Association. 2009. "Best Management Practices for Pharmaceutical Disposal." www.avma.org/issues/policy/pharmaceutical_disposal.asp.

Borgman, Wes. 2007. "Profit and the In-House Pharmacy." *Trends*, March/April, 73–75.

Boss, Nan. 2003. *The Client Education Notebook: Customized Client Education Materials to Use in Your Own Practice*. Vol. 2, *Medical and Medication Information Sheets*. Lincoln, NE: AVLS-PetCom.

Cook, Colleen, and Wendy Meyers. 2003. "How to Price Prescriptions for Profit." *Trends*, August/September, 41.

Fish, Sandra. 2001–2002. "The Price Is Right." *Trends*, December/January, 21–23.

Fritz, Kathy. 2007. "Take the Guesswork out of Inventory." *NAVC Clinician's Brief*, May, 36.

Glassman, Gary I. 2008. "We Have Lots of Inventory: So What's Wrong with That?" *Proceedings of the Central Veterinary Conference*, August 1. See http://veterinarycalendar.dvm 360.com/avhc/Veterinary+technicians/We-have-lots-of-inventory-So-whats-wrong-with-that/ArticleStandard/Article/detail/572690.

Janes, Erika Rasmusson. 2010. "8 Secrets of Inventory Success." *Firstline*, October 1. http://veterinaryteam.dvm360.com/firstline/Veterinary+managers/8-secrets-of-inventory-success/ArticleStandard/Article/detail/690732.

Opperman, Mark. 2009. "Give Your Practice an Inventory Intervention." *Veterinary Economics*, March 1.

Siebert, Phil. 2008. "How to Dispose of Leftover Medications Safely." *Veterinary Economics*, October 1.

Snyder, Gerald. 2000. "Expect 40 Percent Pharmacy Profit." *DVM Newsmagazine*, March.

Whitford, Ron. 2002. "Getting Control of Your Inventory." *Veterinary Forum*, May.

MEDICATION INFORMATION SHEET

All medications can cause side effects in some patients. Fortunately, side effects are usually rare or mild.

The medication ...., which has been prescribed for your pet, is considered to be safe and efficacious for your pet's condition. However, the side effects checked are possible with this medication:

- ☐ Drowsiness
- ☐ Diarrhea
- ☐ Liver damage
- ☐ Hyperactivity/restlessness
- ☐ Increased appetite
- ☐ Panting

- ☐ Nausea/lack of appetite
- ☐ Allergic reaction
- ☐ Kidney damage
- ☐ Increased water consumption/urination
- ☐ Anemia with overdosage or long-term use
- ☐ Other ....

Additional warnings or notations about this medication:

- ☐ Give with food
- ☐ Give on an empty stomach
- ☐ Do not give with dairy products
- ☐ Shake well

- ☐ Keep refrigerated
- ☐ Refill when empty
- ☐ Do not give same day as heartworm pill
- ☐ Wear gloves to administer

- ☐ Do not stop giving medication without consulting us
- ☐ Give until gone—stopping medication too soon can lead to relapse
- ☐ Recheck blood/urine/stool testing is needed in .... days/weeks
- ☐ Do not give along with ....
- ☐ Do not give to animals with a history of seizures or epilepsy
- ☐ Not FDA approved for this purpose or in this species of animal, but is considered to be safe and is commonly used
- ☐ Other ....

QUESTIONING YOUR CLIENTS

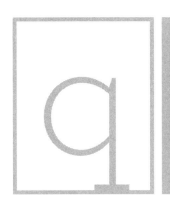

Sometimes, instead of providing information, you will be gathering information from the client. This takes good interviewing and listening skills as well as good note-taking. Getting the pet's history and finding out about its symptoms are essential in good veterinary care, as it is this information that allows the veterinarian to diagnose problems, determine risk factors, and decide on the correct treatment plan. In this section you will learn how to be a sort of investigative reporter for the veterinarians at your clinic, asking the right questions and reporting the answers to them in a concise format.

If you don't have history forms or templates in your hospital, your team can work together to develop some. These can outline the specific questions needed for a given presentation, such as vomiting, and can even allow you to choose from standard or common answers. This makes getting a history faster and more accurate. History forms can either be set up as templates in electronic medical records or printed out as paper forms. At the end of this section there are two sample templates: one for taking a history on upper respiratory signs and the other for gastrointestinal problems. The second one is in "SOAP" format, a standardized method of getting a history. The acronym refers to the fact that you are obtaining *subjective* information, and then going on to fill in the *objective* information, which is the data you collect from the examination and any test procedures that are done. Then comes the *assessment*—which refers to the diagnosis—and finally the *plan* for treating the illness.

Different members of the practice team will handle different aspects of this process. An assistant may obtain the subjective information, and then a technician may handle some of the objective data collection. The veterinarian does the exam to determine what objective information to gather and the assessment to develop the plan, with support from the rest of the team to help educate the client and provide follow-up for his or her instructions.

> **Listen to the client.**

If you are a member of the team who obtains patient histories and asks about current symptoms, be sure to look at and think about any information the team already should be aware of, then ask for clarification. For example, you can say, "Is he still eating Science Diet?" "Is he still on a heartworm preventive?" "Are you giving him any aspirin when he gets sore?" "Are you still using the glucosamine supplement we gave you last time?" "Is there anything else your dog receives besides what you have already listed?"

Clients often don't consider heartworm and flea preventives, aspirin, nutraceuticals, vitamins, and herbal products to be "medicine." You need to ask specific, pointed questions in order to obtain information about these products.

While obtaining information from the client, be sure you are making eye contact, showing empathy, and following the trail of the description the owner is giving you. The history-taking process is like sending a lot of information down a funnel, narrowing it down to a stream of relevant facts that can be used to plan the next steps in diagnosis. While you are doing this, you must not lose sight of the fact that the client may be stressed or anxious and is looking to you for support.

Clients are usually more than happy to answer questions regarding their pets. It's up to you to ask the right ones, to record the answers faithfully, and to follow the path the answers lead you down.

In general, you want to ask simple but open-ended questions. It is important to frame them to get a description, not a "yes" or "no." Avoid asking "why." This question provokes defensiveness and guilt. For example, you would not want to say, "Why did you let him eat that bratwurst if you knew it might make him sick?" Don't ask, "Did you know that chicken bones could be hazardous?" Instead, try to get the client to describe and clarify. Good questions include "Tell me about what happened . . ." "What happened next?" "What thoughts did you have when . . . ?" and "Tell me more about . . ." For some questions, it can be useful to explain why you are asking them. For example, when taking a history, you might say, "Have you noticed Ralphie drinking or urinating more than usual? These are important to notice because diseases such as diabetes and kidney failure will cause these signs," or "Have you noticed any blood or mucous in the stool? This might indicate a problem in the colon and not the small intestine."

Asking smart questions and explaining them to the client involves him or her in your thought process. Remember that the clients are paying money for your expertise, and they appreciate it when you share information that helps them understand their pet and clues them in on what to look for. This helps you get better answers, too, because the client comes to understand that there are good reasons for each question.

When asking questions about routine care, it is important to be diplomatic. Don't make it sound as if you are accusing the client of taking poor care of the pet. When you ask clients what they are feeding the pet, for example, and they name some cheap brand of food, don't say, "Oh, you must be a cheapskate, Mr. Foster." Instead, say, "We don't recommend that brand of food because it may not have the level of nutrition Buster needs to stay healthy. Don't be fooled into thinking all pet foods are alike. The higher-priced brands usually do give you much better nutritional value for your dollar."

As a veterinary technician or veterinary assistant, you should ask about the pet's lifestyle and care each time it is brought in for its annual exam. Point out to the client—and then later to a doctor—areas that may be of concern. These questions prepare the owner to talk about these important issues later with the veterinarian. For example, if a client says "yes" when you have asked whether the pet has dry skin, you could say, "Oh, the doctor will want to talk to you about that. We may want to put Lizzy on a special diet or vitamin supplement." If you notice the pet has tartar on its teeth, you might say, "I see some tartar on Lizzy's teeth. The doctor will want to discuss that with you. Are you able to brush her teeth?"

Remember, it takes five repetitions before any new piece of information is heard and responded to. If the client hears the same message from the veterinary technician, the doctor, and the client relations specialist, he or she is much more likely to agree to Lizzy's dental cleaning.

One of the most difficult things in client relations is learning to actually listen to clients' answers once you have asked them questions. Learn not only to ask the right questions, but also to listen to the answers. Too many times, we jump ahead and start thinking about the next question, failing to pay attention to what the client is saying. Another trap is avoiding certain questions because you are afraid of what the client's answer or response will be. Just because the client is crabby doesn't mean the pet shouldn't get the chance to have that senior screen or ECG done.

> **Learn not only to ask the right questions, but also to listen to the answers.**

Whenever you advise a client that a test, procedure, or medication is needed by the pet, it is imperative that you get a clear "yes" or "no" before proceeding. This means asking questions such as "Is this the treatment plan you want to follow for Scruffy?" "When would you like to schedule the dental cleaning?" or "Do you want to have us do the senior testing we talked about along with the heartworm test, Ms. Costas?" Then you must stop and wait for the client's answer. Do not fill the awkward silence that may follow with disclaimers, explanations, or unnecessary waffling. This only confuses and distracts the client from making a decision and makes the question—and thus the recommended care—seem less important.

Whatever the client's reply, record it clearly on the record (e.g., "senior testing refused at this time"). Then Ms. Costas cannot come back later when Scruffy becomes ill with chronic renal failure and say that you never asked about the test.

A note-taking system recommended by veterinary practice management consultant Dr. Tom Catanzaro works well. This system focuses on recording whether the client has accepted or declined procedures. After each service listed on the patient record as recommended, include a small box. If the client accepts the recommendation, put an "X" in the box, which means the service was performed. If the client says, "No, I don't want that done," put an "R" in the box for "refused the service." If the client says, "Not today, but maybe next time," put a "D" in the box for "deferred until later." If the owner defers a service until a particular time, such as next month or at the next visit, note this next to the box with the "D" in it. If you recommend something over the phone or for a different day, and the owner makes an appointment to have it done, mark an "A" in the box to indicate that he or she made the appointment. In my paperless practice I have templates with drop-down menus for these same common answers, instead of using boxes and handwritten letters.

This system of abbreviation saves some of the time and effort that can be spent writing things on the record. You might also put a dollar sign after the box to signify that the reason the client refused or deferred a service was the cost.

You must be sure you know why the owner refused the procedure or test. You cannot clear up misconceptions on the part of the client about the cost, risks, or benefits if you don't know what is stopping him or her from saying "yes." You can ask, "Is there a particular reason you don't wish to schedule the neuter today, Ms. Hays?" "Are you worried about the anesthesia?" or "Do you understand what will happen to Cuddles if the surgery is not done soon?" If you get a "no" answer from a client, be sure it is not because of a misconception or misunderstanding about what the test or procedure entails.

Don't get discouraged by a few "no" answers and give up on asking questions. A good salesperson, whether he or she is selling health care or vacuum cleaners, needs to focus on the next sale in a positive way and not dwell on the previous refusals. Each occasion is a new opportunity to educate clients and provide expert care for their pets.

> **The entire team must be great communicators!**

Sometimes, clients can be stubborn, mean, or downright ignorant. You don't have any clients like these, do you? Of course you do! Their comments and interactions with you can sometimes make your job both difficult and challenging. Keeping perspective and a sense of humor about your work is helpful. Support and console other team members in their efforts to communicate with clients as well. At least you're not doing it alone. Every member of a veterinary team goes through the same thing and would appreciate what you go through on the job! Realize that even in the best practices, there are clients who will test all your patience and communication skills.

RESOURCE

Catanzaro, Thomas. 1996. *Building the Successful Veterinary Practice,* vol. 2: *Programs and Procedures*. Golden, CO: Catanzaro and Associates. See Chapter 3 on "Medical Records."

SAMPLE FORM/TEMPLATE: TAKING A HISTORY FOR A PET WITH UPPER RESPIRATORY SIGNS

1. How long has the pet been coughing/sneezing, etc.?
2. How often is it doing these things?
3. If it is sneezing, what does the nasal discharge look like? (Clear is often allergy or viral infection; green or yellow is more likely bacterial infection; blood may indicate a foreign body or tumor.)
4. If pet is coughing, is the cough productive and producing mucous, or dry and hacking?
5. Are the eyes mattery, squinting, or closed? If there has been discharge, what color is it?
6. Is the pet breathing normally, or with effort, noise, or discomfort?
7. Is the pet still eating and drinking normally?
8. Is the pet listless or maintaining its usual activities? Have you noticed if the pet tires easily?
9. Has the pet been around other animals that were ill, or has it been boarded, groomed, or housed with other pets?
10. If the patient is new, when were the last vaccinations? Is it on any medications?
11. Is the pet on a heartworm preventive?
12. Are there any other recent changes associated with the symptoms, such as a new pet in the house, woodstove or fireplace being used, new carpet, exposure to cigarette or cigar smoke?
13. Are there any other signs or symptoms you've noticed, such as drinking or urinating more frequently, weakness, gagging, vomiting?

SAMPLE FORM/TEMPLATE: GASTROINTESTINAL (GI) SYSTEM HISTORY

GI SOAP for .... Date .... Wt. .... Client # ....

Subjective: Vomiting is acute/chronic.   Diarrhea is acute/chronic.
Previous bloodwork/fecal ....
Current regular diet .... For how long? ....
Meals per day .... Treats or snacks? ....
When did the vomiting/diarrhea start? ....
How many times/how often has the pet had vomiting/diarrhea? ....
What did the vomit look like?   Food: Always   Just initially   Digested   Undigested   Tube-shaped   Foam
    Clear fluid   Green/yellow   Fluid/bile   Blood   Other ....
If chronic, time/hours after eating: Varies   On empty stomach   Morning/evening
    Usually .... hrs. after meal
What does the stool look like?   Don't know/None   Normal   Hard   Soft/Pudding   Runny/Watery   Blood
    Mucous   Worms seen ....   Leaves/Sticks/Hair   Green/Black/Brown/Yellow
    Other ....
Does the pet strain during/after passing stool?   Y   N   Don't know
When and what did the pet eat last?   Don't know   Eating normally   As follows:
....
When did the pet drink last? ....   Don't know   Normal   Excessive   Small amounts
    Not drinking   Vomiting water
Is the pet on any medication? ....
Other symptoms noted: Lethargic   PU/PD   No urine   Weak   Panting
    Coughing/retching/gagging/sneezing   Bloated   Other: ....
    ....
Possible causes: Ate garbage/dead animal/bones/missing toy/string or
    other items ....
Any other factors?   Ran away   Outside unsupervised   New food
    Change in household ....
Hx of hepatitis/IBD/pancreatitis/SIBO?   Other ....

Objective: T ....   HR ....   RR ....   CRT ....   Skin turgor: N   Slow   Very slow
MM: Normal   Moist   Dry/tacky   Pigmented Pink/Pale/Dark/Bluish   Jaundiced   Excess saliva
Mouth/Throat: Can't examine   Normal   Pharyngitis   Tonsillitis   FB ....
Abd. Palp.:   Normal   Too fat   Tense   Painful cranial/caudal/throughout   Swollen liver/spleen
    Peritoneal fluid   Bladder full/empty/blocked/stones   Kidneys small/Rt. Lt.   Kidneys enlarged/Rt. Lt.
Stool in colon: Y   N   Hard/constipated
Gas/Fluid in bowel   Thickened bowel   Mass/Other: ....

Other systems normal? (eyes, ears, skin, H & L, etc.): Normal ....
....
Thyroid nodule: Pet is   Normal wt.   Thin   Overweight   Obese   Painful   Depressed   Dehydrated

Assessment or Diagnosis/Primary Ruleouts: Colitis   Constipation   Enteritis   Esophagitis/stricture
FB/Linear   Food allergy/IBD   Gastritis   GDV   Giardia/Parasites   Hepatitis/Fatty liver   Hyperthyroid
Megaesoph   Neoplasia   Open   Pancreatitis/EPI   Parvo/Corona   Pyometra   Renal   SIBO
Urinary blockage   Other: ....
Prognosis: Grave   Poor   Fair   Guarded   Good   Excellent
Recc. Referral to: ....   For: ....

Plan: CBC out/in   Chem panel out/in   GI panel (cobalamin, folate, PLI/TLI)   PLI out/in
      T4 TLI Bile acids/P & P Draw blood & hold ....
Blood test results: ....
....
Fecal float/cyt/dir/Gia Ag results: Campyl.   Clost.   Coccidia   Giardia   Hooks   Rounds   Spirochetes
      Tapes   Whips   Other: ....
Enema(s) ....   X-rays   EH/O. to wait   Abd. Lat/VD   Chest Lat/VD   Barium swallow/series   OG tube
Sedative inj. cc   ....IM/SQ
X-ray results: NSF ....
Surgery: Endoscopy   Enterotomy   FB removal   Gastrotomy   Laparoscopy   Laparotomy
      Relieve urinary obstruction   U/S   Other ....
Hospitalize   IV fluids   SQ fluids   cc LRS
Antinausea meds: ....
Antibiotics: ....
Other medications: ....
Oral meds: In hospital: ....
To go home: ....
Diet   NPO .... hrs.   Water in .... hrs.   Food in.................. hrs.
Type/brand: ....   Canned/dry   Amount ....
For how long? ....
Then mix with reg. diet for ....   Syringe feed? ....
Other instructions: ....
Recheck: Fecal float 10 days/6 weeks/other ....   Fecal cytology   7   10   14   days
Other recheck testing: ....   Call back in: 1   2   4   7   days
Handouts given: GI care/pancreatitis/ ....
Discharge instructions given by: ....   Diagnostic code ....   Estimate: ....

Notes:

RISK MANAGEMENT

Much of our work in veterinary medicine hinges on the concept of reducing risk. Vaccinations reduce the risk of infectious diseases, parasite preventives reduce the risk of parasites, senior screening reduces the risk that we will fail to detect a disease process early, and so on. In fact, most of the topics covered in this book are about risks we can educate clients about, such as behavior problems, dental disease, and cancer. Client education follows risk assessment and management. We teach the clients about topics that pertain to their pet—those illnesses for which the pet is at risk.

Most clients visit us only a few times a year, and we have a limited amount of time during each of those visits to educate and inform them. In order to make the most of the time that we have, it's important to prioritize, and that means taking a pet's risk factors and disease exposure into account when deciding what to focus on for each visit.

Educating clients about the health risks their pets have is best done in stages. We start with risks that every pet has, such as for infectious diseases and parasites, and then work our way up toward the more individualized risks that depend on a pet's genetics and lifestyle. This is the same process we use in puppy and kitten visits: We begin with vaccinations and parasite control and work up to dental care and microchipping. A hunting dog and an indoor cat both have a risk for distemper virus, but in other ways the things that would be most likely to damage their health are very different. You must learn how to prioritize accordingly.

There are several ways to go about prioritizing pets' risks and needs. One way is to think about the frequency of diseases, categorizing them as "most common," "somewhat common," and "not very common," and then focus on those that are most common.

> Think of yourself as a teacher.

You wouldn't spend much time educating clients about a disease you only see a few times a year, or one a particular patient is unlikely to ever encounter. You'd spend the valuable time you had with clients at wellness visits to talk about common things. You would want to incorporate these topics into a broad educational plan. A simple way to do this is to choose one or two topics to focus on per year so you can educate every client about them. Examples would be dental care and obesity.

This is as simple as putting a handout in every file before the appointment so you remember to discuss the topic with clients and send them home with written information. Preparing and preloading your patient files ahead of each visit is a very important step. Have a system. If this is the year the clinic wants to educate every client on dental disease, load a dental brochure in every file. If you have already taught your clients about dental care, then maybe you could develop a cancer-prevention handout instead.

For older pets, have a senior-care program that addresses disease risks for older pets and how to test for them. Chronic kidney disease is rare in young pets but common in older ones, so you might bring up that topic for owners of older pets, in addition to dentistry and obesity. Chemistry and thyroid testing, urinalysis and urine protein, and blood pressure testing and screening for eye diseases such as dry eye (KCS) would all be topics for discussion, depending on the species and breed of the pet.

Because there are more topics to cover for seniors, and you are adding them to the basic care needs you already have to discuss, it's wise to schedule 10 extra minutes for senior pet appointments. The doctor can be teaching the client about the importance of wellness testing while the technician is drawing the blood sample or taking a blood pressure reading.

If a pet comes in with other problems or priorities, then focus your client-education efforts on those things. For example, if your focus for client education this year is dental care, but your patient is a senior pet who comes in with severe arthritis and infected ears, maybe you wouldn't get to the dental disease information at that visit. You would instead note in the file to go over it at the recheck when the pet is doing better. But having an overall plan for all patients helps you to keep your focus.

The second way to prioritize risk is by seriousness of problem. In this scheme, those with a higher risk for death or illness would be at the top of the list. The categories would be (1) diseases and problems that could be fatal; (2) diseases or problems that could cause pain, suffering, or chronic damage; and (3) diseases or problems that could cause inconvenience or mild illness.

For this system of categorizing risks, you need to take into account breed and lifestyle. The problem that may be the biggest health risk for one patient may not be the same one that is the biggest for another patient. Instead of dentistry or obesity, for example, it may be that the dog goes to a groomer but isn't being vaccinated against kennel cough.

Try using a questionnaire to find out what you need to address with clients. When each animal comes in for its annual or semiannual exam, ask the client a set of questions about the pet. Use the answers the client gives you to determine which services to recommend. For instance, asking whether a dog goes to see a groomer regularly might prompt you to recommend Bordetella vaccination. Asking whether a cat is allowed outdoors tells you about that pet's risk for feline leukemia. You can learn who's using ineffective grocery-store flea products, who should be cleaning the cocker's ears but isn't, and who would be interested in learning to brush the pet's teeth.

Breed-specific wellness is the next big leap for educating clients if you already covered all the basics. Breed tendencies for disease can jump right to the top of your "diseases or problems that could be fatal" list in some cases. For example, cardiomyopathy is common and deadly in boxers but occurs later and in a milder form in some other breeds. The more common and the more severe the risk, the more you need to talk about it early and often. For a boxer owner, you would make this risk, and annual electrocardiogram (ECG) screening, a big priority, but for a Dalmatian you would choose something else to talk about, such as bladder stones. Instead of ECG screening, you would discuss feeding the Dalmatian a special diet and performing an annual urinalysis. Think about and discuss scripts for breed-related testing if you want to educate clients in a particular area. For example: "Boxers are at risk for serious heart problems. The doctor will talk to you about ECG screening . . ."

Genetics influence what we test and educate for because 40 percent of purebred dogs have genetic defects. Close to 500 canine and 300 feline genetic diseases have been described to date. Disorders caused by a single genetic defect can be more easily diagnosed and treated than those involving more complex genetic patterns, such as hip dysplasia. More genetic tests are becoming available all the time.

A few genetic problems are evident from the start or by the time a puppy is old enough to leave its mother and go into a new home. Many, however, develop or become evident as a puppy or kitten grows, or later as it ages. Some of these genetic diseases can be tested for in ways that enable veterinarians to diagnose them early and begin intervention. Some simply require awareness on the part of the owner as to what to watch for and when to call the veterinarian.

> **Close to 500 canine and 300 feline genetic diseases have been described to date. Disorders caused by a single genetic defect can be more easily diagnosed and treated than those involving more complex genetic patterns, such as hip dysplasia. More genetic tests are becoming available all the time.**

One example we are all familiar with is hip dysplasia. For large and at-risk breeds it is important to screen dogs for it and to educate owners about arthritis diagnosis and treatment. Liver disease is another example because it is also more common in certain breeds. For some breeds it is useful to test bile acids when the puppy is young. For others, hepatitis screening should be done when the dog is middle-aged or older.

Collect information that will allow you to make good recommendations for the individual pet. These recommendations may affect diet, exercise routine, exposure to other pets, and so on. Evaluate risks and record them. Then educate the client about the risks you've identified for that patient.

When educating a client about a pet's risks, choose no more than three topics to touch on, and one or two of them that you will spend more time on or reinforce with written information that the client can take home. When discussing topics with pet owners, remember that they often do not perceive things the way we do. To you it's another patient—to them it's a family member. Any bleeding, swelling, lump, or disease symptom in a pet may seem frightening to a client. Clients also don't want to think about their pets becoming old or sick, so you need to talk about keeping the pet healthy rather than focusing on the negative aspects of disease and aging.

Keep in mind that this may be the twentieth client you've seen today, but it may be the client's only visit all year. You need to sound cheerful, positive, and enthusiastic and strive to make learning about pet care fun, even if you are tired or distracted. What do you want each client to comply with? You need to find out what the client's and pet's needs are and then prioritize those needs. Document them in your medical records. What are the most important things, and what can wait until next time?

Remember to use *value statements* (see the "Over-the-Counter Sales" section). Praise the client for doing things right, when possible. Most of all, remember that the guidance you give clients on reducing the risks you've identified will determine, in great part, how long and how happily a pet will live. Use the time you have with your clients wisely. (See also "Yearly Exam and Senior Health-Care Recommendations" for more information about educating clients during office visits and offering consistent care.)

At the end of this section is an example of a form that team members can use while interviewing clients to help determine risk factors for a particular pet. It is not intended as a handout to clients. Instead, its purpose is to ensure that the interviewer remembers to ask the questions included. You can adapt it to your practice by adding questions that you believe will be helpful for determining risks for the pets you see.

RESOURCES

Boss, Nan. 2010. *Canine Assessments and Genetic Testing Cheat Sheet*. San Antonio, TX: VetThink. This book lays out a wellness and prevention plan for each of over 100 dog breeds.

DVM360, www.dvm360.com. DVM360 has a number of items useful for performing risk assessments. From the "Business Center" menu, choose "Patient Care" or "Client Handouts" and look for "Canine Lifestyle Review" and "Feline Lifestyle Review," "Dog Lifestyle Survey," and "Technician In-Room Checklist." Under "Patient Care" you'll also find "Compliance Review Form" and one entitled "Catch Clients with Review Form."

Gough, Alex, and Alison Thomas. 2004. *Breed Predispositions to Disease in Dogs and Cats*. Oxford: Blackwell.

Jevring, Caroline, and Tom Catanzaro. 1999. *Healthcare of the Well Pet*. Philadelphia: W. B. Saunders.

VetThink, www.vetthinkinc.com. This company publishes the Genesis Breed-Specific Health Care Wellness Books, a series of booklets and handouts on each of 75 different breeds, to give to clients. Each breed booklet includes a chart of services recommended for that breed at every age.

———. 2003. *The Client Education Notebook: Customized Client Education Materials to Use in Your Own Practice*. Lincoln, NE: AVLS-PetCom. Volume 1 includes handout sets for puppies, kittens, adult cats and dogs, and senior cats and dogs. These materials focus on wellness and preventive care. A CD in Microsoft Word lets you customize them to your practice. Volume 2 contains medication information sheets and a variety of client handouts on topics not covered elsewhere. Some are about symptoms that need to be worked up (vs. diseases or diagnoses). This set also lists each breed and the genetic problems for which that breed is at risk.

RISK ASSESSMENT QUESTIONNAIRE

Pet's Name .... Date ....

What is the pet's primary role in the family? (hunting dog, family pet, barn cat, breeding, therapy/assistant dog, etc.) ....

If you are not brushing your pet's teeth, would you like us to show you how? ....

What medications is your pet currently taking? ....

Do you give any supplements, herbs, or over-the-counter medications to your pet? ....

Does your pet have any lumps, warts, or skin lesions?   Y   N
   Describe ....

Does your pet have any behavioral problems you wish to discuss with the doctor?   Y   N
   Describe ....

Any other problems or concerns? (vomiting, diarrhea, cough, urinary symptoms, etc.)   Y   N
   Describe ....

(If the client is not buying from us) Do you use flea or tick control products on your pet?   Y   N
   If so, what do you use and how often? ....

Does your cat go outside?   Y   N   Loose or leashed? ....

Do you travel with your pet, or do you plan on moving soon (need health cert.?)?   Y   N

Do you take your dog hunting, hiking, or camping?   Y   N

How often do you bathe your pet, and what products do you use? ....

Does your dog go swimming?   Y   N   If so, how often? ....

Does your dog go to a groomer or dog park, or board at a kennel?   Y   N

Do you clean your pet's ears regularly?   Y   N   Trim its nails?   Y   N

Do you plan on adding cats or kittens to your household within the next year?   Y   N
   (If so, discuss FeLV, URI, introducing a new cat, etc.)

Do you plan on adding dogs or puppies to your household within the next year?   Y   N
   (If so, discuss prepurchase counseling)

Have you noticed any of the following signs in your pet? (Give a value statement)

- [ ] Loss of house training or litter-box avoidance   - [ ] Increased thirst or urination
- [ ] Excessive panting/breathing changes   - [ ] Changes in activity level   - [ ] Increased stiffness
- [ ] Less interaction with the family   - [ ] Confusion or disorientation   - [ ] Decreased hearing
- [ ] Decreased responsiveness   - [ ] Changes in sleeping patterns   - [ ] Skin and hair coat changes
- [ ] Weight change   - [ ] Altered appetite   - [ ] Difficulty jumping up   - [ ] Difficulty climbing steps
- [ ] Other ....

SURGERY AND ANESTHESIA

Nothing strikes fear into a client's heart more than the two words "anesthesia" and "surgery." Everybody seems to know someone who had a pet die when under anesthesia. Most clients think the risks are far greater than they actually are. It is the veterinary team's duty to reassure the client and put those fears to rest, especially if the fear is preventing the owner from scheduling a needed procedure for his or her pet.

Safer anesthetic drugs, anesthetic monitors, and the availability of presurgical testing, such as blood chemistries and electrocardiograms (ECGs), have made anesthesia much safer today than it was in years past. The risk of problems from the anesthesia or surgery is usually far lower than the risk of not performing a needed procedure. Tell your clients that their pets will probably live much healthier lives if the needed care is provided in a timely fashion.

The risk of problems from the anesthesia or surgery is usually far lower than the risk of not performing a needed procedure.

To reassure clients, you can say: "We'll take the best possible care of her" or "Dr. Smith is a skilled surgeon. You can count on him to do a great job for Fluffy." Another good comment is: "Fluffy will feel so much better after this is done!" If a client seems worried, ask, "Do you have any questions or concerns about the surgery?" And when the surgery is completed and you call the client with an update, let him or her know right away that all is well: "She's still sleepy, but everything went just fine," and "I'm looking at her right now, and she's already sitting up," are both good phrases to memorize and use.

When discussing surgery, you must make sure clients understand what will be done and how it will be done. They will want to know how long the pet will stay in the hospital, what kind of care it will need when it goes home, and whether the pet will be in pain. (As a general rule, if a procedure would be pain-

SPAYING AND NEUTERING

a pet's spay or neuter surgery may be the only major procedure that pet ever undergoes in your hospital. Even though we take routine procedures for granted, there are risks involved that both you and the client should be aware of. Take the time to carefully explain what the pet will need to have done and the safety precautions the medical and technical staff will be taking. Be careful to explain the pain management protocol as well.

Clients will often ask you whether spaying or neutering will make their pets fat. These surgeries do change metabolism and appetite. However, that doesn't mean the pet has to become overweight. It also depends on the pet's activity level and how much he or she is fed. Owners should be warned that they will need to be much more careful with the amounts they feed their pets after spaying and neutering to help avoid obesity in the future. Tell clients specifically how much to feed their pets and warn them not to go by the directions on the pet-food container—these are almost always too generous.

You can say to the owner: "Spaying will change your pet's metabolism and she will no longer need as much food to grow or to maintain her body weight. Watch her weight closely over the next few months, as you may need to decrease the amount of food you are feeding her. It is much easier to prevent excessive weight gain than it is to get the

ful for a person, it will be painful for the pet.) If the pet will need medication to be administered when it gets home, such as antibiotics or pain medication, the client should be informed ahead of time. The client should get an accurate estimate and updates on any additional charges that accrue.

Questions about spaying and neutering are common. You will need to learn some basics about these procedures so that you can answer clients' questions about when to have them performed and what happens during and after surgery. The benefits of spaying or neutering pets, the safety of the anesthesia and the surgery itself, presurgery options, and prices for these procedures are all questions you need to know how to answer. Noninvasive surgery options are becoming more common, so you may need to learn about those, too. Any questions you can't answer should be referred to a team member with expertise in that area.

---

pounds off once they are there, and being overweight has serious health consequences for your pet. We will call you in six weeks to ask you to bring her in for a weight check. That way, if she starts to get too heavy we will catch it early."

Clients will also ask whether spaying or neutering can change a pet's personality. Reassure them that although it's true that a pet's personality can change, it's usually for the better. You can tell them that neutered pets tend to be more focused on their owners and much less likely to roam and fight. And when they are less likely to roam, they are less likely to be hit by cars.

In addition, pets that are spayed or neutered live longer, on average, than those that are not. Spaying or neutering can reduce the risk of some diseases and infections that affect the reproductive organs.

Some pet owners are interested in breeding their pets, and for them, spaying or neutering is not an option. For most pet owners, spaying or neutering is the best choice. There are too many unwanted cats and dogs in animal shelters that end up being euthanized. In addition, having the surgery done means that the pet owner will not have to deal with heat cycles, cats that spray in the house, and other problems that come with having a pet that is not spayed or neutered. (See "Benefits of Spaying and Neutering" text box for more information.)

Owners of pets entering the hospital for surgery or dental care can be prepped ahead of time with presurgery letters that explain the procedure and the process involved. A sample presurgery handout is provided at the end of this section (see "What You Need to Know Before Your Pet's Upcoming Surgery").

Send your letter out seven to 10 days before a scheduled procedure, or give one to the client in the office if the surgery is imminent. You can have several versions of this form if you want the information to be more specific. One would be for dog spays or neuters, for example, outlining the surgical risks in general, the medication the veterinarian is recommending for pain control, and a set of options and prices. Options can include microchipping or tattoos, blood testing, fluid therapy, pain medication, ECG, breed-specific testing, and many other things, depending on the individual pet. Do not bombard

BENEFITS OF SPAYING AND NEUTERING

Some clients intend to breed their pets. Once they have expressed that desire, obviously you are not going to push the spaying and neutering procedures on them. However, for most clients the primary goal is to get them to spay or neuter their pets. Most clients already plan to have the surgery done, but others need a lot of convincing. You need to be prepared to tell them about the benefits of the procedure to help them make the decision to have the procedure done at the appropriate time.

You can explain, for example, that spaying or neutering helps to prevent some of the later problems that pets can have. The biggies that spaying prevents are pyometra (severe infection in the uterus) and mammary (breast) tumors. Most intact females will eventually develop one or the other or both. Spaying before the first heat cycle nearly eliminates the risk of mammary cancer, and spaying at any age removes the risk of pyometra. Ovarian or uterine tumors, Brucellosis, and transmissible venereal warts are other problems seen in intact females, though these are less common.

As with pyometra and mammary tumors in females, the risks of benign prostatic hypertrophy and perianal tumors are very high in older intact males. Prostatic cancer can occur in neutered or intact males, but testicular cancer, of course, is not a risk once a dog is castrated. In intact male cats, roaming, fighting, and contagious diseases such as feline leukemia (FeLV) and feline immunodeficiency virus (FIV) are common. (Nineteen percent of cats with abscesses or bite wounds have FeLV or FIV; see the FeLV/FIV guidelines at www.aafponline.org.)

In both dogs and cats that have not been spayed or neutered, behaviors such as territorial marking/spraying, aggression, and roaming are frequent problems. Intact male dogs are a minority of the total dog population but account for the majority of dogs hit by cars. According to Spay/Neuter Your Pet (SNYP), an Oregon-based spay/neuter service, four out of every five dogs hit by a car are unneutered males.

Last, of course, there's pet overpopulation. Simply put, there are too many pets. Eight million to 10 million lost and unwanted dogs and cats enter animal shelters every year in the United States, and 4 million to 6 million of them are euthanized. As long as there are not homes for all of them, any animal added to the population, for whatever reason, helps feed companion-animal overpopulation and contributes to the massive number of animals in shelters. It's not just a problem of mixed breeds, either: Twenty-five percent of dogs at shelters are purebred.

Repetition is important here. Keep mentioning the importance of the surgery to the health of the pet. Tell an anecdote or two about pregnancies that end in the death or illness of the mother or puppies, or tell clients about a case where an unspayed male dog caused lots of behavior problems or repeatedly ran away. If they think they want kittens or want to be able to see kittens born, be sure you tell Mom that she's the one who will probably have to take care of the mess, find good homes, and shoo away the yowling and spraying tomcats outside the house.

What really seem to motivate owners to have their pets spayed or neutered are things that impact their own lives, not the pets' lives. Things such as the pet lifting its leg or spraying in the house; messy or noisy heat cycles; male dogs hanging around the house or going after females down the street; the money and time that must be spent to put ads in the paper and entertain prospective buyers of puppies; and all the other hassles of breeding ultimately get clients to spay or neuter. That's what you have to emphasize and discuss every time the client comes to the clinic.

clients with choices on the morning of the surgery that they haven't already heard about. Clients are often nervous about leaving their pet with you, may be in a hurry to get to work, and are easily distracted. If you send the letter to the client in the mail, you will also be getting in one of those five repetitions needed to make a sale.

Also include a separate page in this mailing that explains anesthesia procedures at your clinic. A sample handout of this type is included at the end of this section (see "Anesthesia and Your Pet"). If the client didn't get one with the last puppy or kitten visit, enclose a brochure about pre-anesthetic blood testing when you mail the presurgery letter.

Write it down!

You might want to have a different letter for cat surgeries. Most cats we see aren't purebreds, so you can leave out the information on breed risk testing. In addition, we often use different anesthetics and pain medications for cats, so you would need to explain those.

If specialized procedures are performed in your clinic, separate versions of the presurgery letter can be created for each one. Informed consent is getting more complicated all the time, as the standard of care and number of available services keep going up.

When these letters are sent ahead of time, clients usually come to the clinic prepared to tell you their decisions. Even if the primary caretaker of the pet isn't the one dropping the pet off for surgery, the decisions have been made, though they may be reported to you by phone or through the person who is bringing the pet in.

On the day of surgery, be sure the owner knows when to call for an update on the pet's condition. A technician or doctor might want to call the owner

Sending the client a text message to say the pet's procedure was a success, and attaching a picture of the pet in recovery (cuddled up to a stuffed animal), is a great extra touch on surgery day.

after the surgery to let him or her know how things went. If problems arise, it is always best for the doctor to call rather than another team member.

Because many clients worry when their pets are in the hospital, give them frequent updates. Sending the client a text message to say the pet's procedure was a success, and attaching a picture of the pet in recovery (cuddled up to a stuffed animal), is a great extra touch on surgery day.

Every pet should go home with a written release form explaining the home care that is needed while it recovers. A typical surgery release form appears at the end of this section (see "Care of Your Pet Following Surgery"). You will need to customize the release for particular surgeries. For example, for spays and neuters, you may want to include a line or two about monitoring for weight gain and decreasing the amount of food after the surgery.

THINGS TO CONSIDER FOR EVERY SURGERY

While the pet is under anesthesia, it is a perfect time to take care of other elective procedures. Remember that you may not have the opportunity again until years from now when the pet needs its teeth cleaned or a lump removed. You can offer microchipping or nail trims, of course, but also think about genetic problems you could screen for at this time. If you neuter a pet at six months of age, it's way too early for OFA hip X-rays, as the hip joints are not mature yet—but performing hip X-rays while the dog is under anesthesia anyway will give you an idea as to whether this pet will have major problems with hip dysplasia later on.

Blood-clotting disorders such as von Willebrand's disease are common in some breeds, so doing a buccal bleeding time (BBT, a quick bleeding test involving a nick on the inside of the animal's lip) before surgery might be indicated in some dogs. Bile acids testing to screen for hepatic microdysplasia or shunting (abnormal blood vessels within or going around the liver) would be indicated for Yorkshire terriers. A careful soft palate exam and resection (cutting back), if needed, could be done for pugs and bulldogs. Think about these things before surgery and discuss them during puppy visits so owners are comfortable with these ideas by the time surgery day rolls around.

> **PAIN-MANAGEMENT TIP**
>
> For every surgery, be careful to explain your pain-management program to the pet owner. Many clients do not understand or recognize signs of pain in their pets and tend to underestimate and undermedicate. There is no reason for an animal to be in pain after a procedure. Many times clients worry way too much about medication side effects and way too little about the risks of untreated pain. Postoperative complication rates are much higher when pets don't receive adequate pain management.

Spend some time with the client at discharge to review the release forms and ensure he or she understands the aftercare needed for the pet. This should be done at a scheduled time in an exam room or other quiet area where the client will not be distracted. The client should be shown any radiographs taken and should receive copies of labwork performed. Technicians or assistants can often perform routine releases, but more complicated cases are usually discharged by the doctor.

Be sure to call the client a day or two after the pet goes home to see how things are going. Most computer systems can flag callbacks for you. A simple system of calling pet owners on the surgery log one or two days before the surgery works well, too. Owners want to know you care about their dog or cat. The extra phone call after the surgery can also help you catch minor problems, such as incision licking, before they become major ones. Many clients will hesitate to call you about a small problem but will worry about it needlessly, or perhaps do the wrong thing to correct it.

It's easy to become blasé about surgical procedures when you see them every day. Clients, however, may be worried. Be sensitive to the owners' concerns and try to make them feel comfortable about the procedures their pets need. Think of how nervous you get when your own pet is under anesthesia. A little handholding and a lot of kindness and personal attention go a long way to reassuring the pet owner after his or her furry family member has undergone a major procedure.

RESOURCES

Abbott Animal Health, www.AbbottAnimalHealthCE.com. Abbott's very informative CE-accredited courses on fluid therapy and anesthesia are offered at this site.

American Association of Feline Practitioners, www.catvets.com. From this site you can link to the AAFP's position statements on early spay and neuter as well as declawing.

DVM360, www.dvm360.com. Here you will find a few useful items for educating clients about surgery topics. Under the "Business Center" menu, choose the "Patient Care" or "Client Handouts" menu to find the client handout "Important Reasons to Spay or Neuter Your Pet" and a "Certificate of Bravery" to award patients after surgery, as well as a post-op care form entitled "My Big Day." For developing scripts to educate clients, look for "Explain the Benefits of Spaying and Neutering Pets."

Gough, Alex, and Alison Thomas. 2004. *Breed Predispositions to Disease in Dogs and Cats*. Oxford: Blackwell.

VetThink, www.vetthinkinc.com. This company publishes the Genesis Breed-Specific Health Care Wellness Books, a series of booklets and handouts on each of 75 different breeds to give to clients. It also offers breed-specific electronic newsletters. Each breed booklet for clients includes a chart of services recommended at different ages specific to the needs of that breed. This includes screening for genetic diseases at the time of spaying or neutering.

WHAT YOU NEED TO KNOW BEFORE YOUR PET'S UPCOMING SURGERY

Many people have questions about various aspects of their pet's surgery, and we hope this handout will help. It also explains the decisions you will need to make before your pet's upcoming surgery.

Is the anesthetic safe?

Today's modern anesthetics and anesthetic monitors have made surgery much safer than in the past. Here at .... Animal Hospital, we do a thorough physical exam on your pet before administering anesthetics to ensure that a fever or other illness won't be a problem. We also adjust the amount and type of anesthetic used depending on the health of your pet. The handout on anesthesia explains this in greater detail.

Pre-anesthetic blood testing is important in reducing the risk of anesthesia. Every pet needs blood testing before surgery to ensure that the liver and kidneys can handle the anesthetic. Even apparently healthy animals can have serious organ system problems that cannot be detected without blood testing. If there is a problem, it is much better to find out about it before it causes anesthetic or surgical complications! Animals that have minor dysfunctions will handle the anesthetic better if they get IV fluids during surgery. If serious problems are detected, surgery can be postponed until the problem is corrected.

The most common cause of unexpected death under anesthesia is an undiagnosed heart problem. An electrocardiogram, or ECG, before and during surgery gives us a heart rhythm strip that will show abnormal heart rhythm or heart enlargement. Even young, apparently healthy pets can have an irregular heartbeat that could be fatal under anesthesia. For senior or ill pets, additional blood tests or X-rays may be required before surgery as well.

For many breeds of dogs, specific testing or procedures may be recommended. For example, Doberman pinschers are prone to a blood-clotting disorder called von Willebrand's disease. This disease can increase the risk of bleeding during or after surgery. Testing the blood's ability to clot properly may be recommended for certain breeds, such as Dobies. Toy breeds are prone to liver dysfunction, so extra liver testing may be needed.

It is important that surgery be done on an empty stomach to reduce the risk of the pet vomiting while under anesthesia and afterward. You will need to withhold food for at least eight hours before surgery. Water can be left out for the pet until the morning of surgery.

Will my pet have stitches?

For many surgeries, we use absorbable sutures underneath the skin. These will dissolve on their own and do not need to be removed. Some surgeries, especially tumor removals, do require skin stitches or staples. With either type of suture, you will need to keep an eye on the incision for swelling or discharge. Most dogs and cats do not lick excessively or chew at the incision, but this is an occasional problem, and you will need to watch for it. If there are skin sutures, these will usually be removed 10 to 14 days after surgery.

You will also need to limit your pet's activity level for a time, and no baths are allowed for the first 10 days after surgery.

Will my pet be in pain?

Anything that causes pain in people can be expected to cause pain in animals. Pets may not show the same symptoms of pain as people do—they do not usually whine or cry—but you can be sure they feel it. We use local anesthetics on the incision site to keep your pet more comfortable for the first few hours after surgery.

Other pain medications needed will depend on the surgery performed. For dogs, we may recommend an oral pain reliever/anti-inflammatory about 24 hours before surgery to lessen the risk of discomfort and swelling. These pills are continued for one to two weeks after the surgery as well. We use newer medications that are less likely than older ones to cause stomach upset and can be given even on the morning of surgery. Please come in at least two days before the scheduled surgery to pick up the medication for your pet.

For years, we have undermedicated cats for pain because cats do not tolerate standard pain medications such as aspirin, ibuprofen, or Tylenol. Recent advances in pain medications have allowed for better pain control in cats than ever before. For some procedures we use a narcotic pain patch. The patch is applied to a small shaved area on the back of the cat's neck and provides continuous pain relief for three to five days. For less severe pain we usually use oral pain medications. Injectable pain medications may also be used on both dogs and cats. We use narcotic patches for some surgeries in dogs as well.

Providing appropriate pain relief is a humane and caring thing to do for your pet. We have a variety of effective medications to choose from to provide the exact amount and type of pain management that are best for your pet.

What other decisions do I need to make?

While your pet is under anesthesia is the ideal time to perform other minor procedures, such as nail trimming, dentistry, ear cleaning, or implanting an identification microchip. Good hip radiographs require anesthesia, so if your dog is a breed or size that might be prone to hip dysplasia, you might want us to take hip X-rays.

We will ask you about these extra procedures when you bring your pet in. If you would like an estimate for these extra services, please call ahead of time. This is especially important if the person dropping the pet off for surgery is not the primary decision-maker for the pet's care.

When you bring your pet in for surgery, you will need 10 to 20 minutes to fill out paperwork and tell us your decisions on the blood testing, ECG screening, and other options. When you pick up your pet after surgery, you can also plan to spend about 10 to 20 minutes to go over your pet's home-care needs.

We will call you the night before your pet's scheduled surgery to confirm your admission time and to answer any questions you might have. In the meantime, please don't hesitate to call us to discuss your pet's health or surgery.

ANESTHESIA AND YOUR PET

Many pet owners worry unnecessarily about anesthesia in their pets. Although anesthesia can never be completely free of risk, today's modern techniques make that risk very small.

The same anesthetic procedures that allow complicated surgeries such as heart and kidney transplants to be performed in humans are used in pets as well. Even very frail animals can usually be anesthetized safely. In general, the risks from not performing a needed procedure, such as dental cleaning or tumor removal, are much higher than the risk from the anesthesia.

We use pre-operative blood tests, electrocardiogram (ECG) screening, and radiographs (X-rays) to help us determine whether a procedure will be safe for your pet before we begin. We require pre-operative blood screening before anesthesia is administered. Even young and apparently healthy animals can have serious organ dysfunctions that are not evident without such testing. Chest X-rays are taken if there is any suspicion of heart or lung disease or cancer.

ECGs are recommended pre-operatively for all pets. An ECG is especially recommended for breeds of cats and dogs that have increased risk for cardiomyopathy, a serious heart condition.

During anesthesia, your pet will be monitored closely throughout the surgery for blood oxygen levels, blood pressure, temperature, heart rate, and heartbeat intensity. The anesthesia is always administered by certified and licensed veterinary technicians or doctors to ensure safety and proper dosing. Intravenous fluids are administered during almost all procedures to maintain blood pressure and hydration during anesthesia.

Through testing, monitoring, and other measures, we will do everything we can to take good care of your pet while it is under anesthesia. Whether it is six weeks old or 16 years old, your pet should be just as perky after recovering from surgery as when it arrived at the hospital. If you have further concerns about anesthesia in your pet, we would be happy to discuss the risks and benefits of any procedure with you and explain the exact protocol that will be used. Please let us know!

CARE OF YOUR PET FOLLOWING SURGERY

Pet's Name ....

Your pet may appear a little uncoordinated and tired when you first take it home. This is normal following surgery. Keep your pet confined and limit exercise for the first 48 hours. If you have any questions, please feel free to call us.

Please report immediately any diarrhea, vomiting, abnormal water drinking or urination, or other symptoms.

- ☐ Report any drainage, injury, or licking of the incision. Keep the incision dry. (No baths for at least seven days following surgery.)
- ☐ Keep all casts and bandages clean and dry. If they do become wet, they must be changed as soon as possible.

Other Instructions ....

....

....

....

Food and Water

Animals confined or having undergone anesthesia tend to drink excessive amounts of water when they first go home. Give small amounts of tepid water every 30 to 60 minutes until the animal's thirst is satisfied.

- ☐ Your animal has been fed today. Feed your pet a regular diet lightly tomorrow and return gradually to normal feeding.
- ☐ Tonight, feed your pet half the regular ration. Return to regular feeding tomorrow.
- ☐ Other diet ....

Future Treatments

- ☐ Please return for a checkup in .... days.
- ☐ Please return to have stitches removed in .... days.

TELEPHONE SKILLS

The telephone is the most important instrument in the hospital. It is the source of nearly all the hospital's business and provides the "first contact" most clients have with the hospital. Good service to the client depends in large part on how you present yourself over the phone. The telephone also helps you to teach. Even the simplest interaction over the phone can allow you to promote your hospital and build rapport with the client.

Entire books have been written on phone etiquette, but here is a brief overview of some tips I've found helpful. Phrases that cannot be said too often are: "Thank you," "You're welcome," "Certainly!" and "I'll be happy to!" Use the client's name often. If you are new at your job, tell the client that up-front—clients will be very understanding when you are slow or unsure if they know the reason. Assure them you will do your best and refer them to someone else if you cannot help them. Likewise, if you are new at the front desk, put on a big badge that says "trainee," and the clients will put up with almost any delay or small error.

Offer clients more information than they ask for. If you are unsure of the answer to a question, look it up or ask someone else. Never give clients misinformation. Offer to call them back or send them literature on the subject if you can't give them an answer immediately.

Never argue with clients. Never talk down to them or sound bored or impatient. If you suspect the caller is trying to sell something, ask, "Is this concerning a pet?" or "May I ask the doctor to return your call?"

When you are dealing with new client calls and requests for prices, grasp the opportunity and make the most of it. Clients don't just call for the price. They will judge you on how friendly you are, how long they waited on hold, and your presentation of the practice. Failure to turn phone shoppers into customers can cost a clinic thousands of dollars each year. One client who stays for 15 years may be worth $5,000 to $15,000. No matter how busy you are, take the time to promote your practice and its services and to send the shopper a brochure or newsletter in the mail. Take the client's name and phone number and call him or her back promptly if you can't spend the time you need at the time of the call.

Value statements work well with phone shoppers (see the "Over-the-Counter Sales" section). For example, when a client calls to ask the price of a dental cleaning for the pet you could say, "The price depends on what level of dental disease is present and what level of care you want for your pet. A dental cleaning involves anesthesia, so we always need to check a blood sample beforehand to make sure the liver and kidney function is adequate to handle the anesthesia. We also recommend an ECG screen for heart function, because pets that die under anesthesia almost always have heart problems. We give IV fluids during the procedure for added safety. The cleaning and polishing of the teeth, and a barrier gel treatment to reduce plaque buildup, are included, as is the day's stay and care in the hospital, the anesthesia, and an antibiotic injection. Any extra services, such as full-mouth X-rays, antibiotics, or extractions that might be necessary would be in addition to the base price of $249.50."

The script is designed to let the client know what is involved in the procedure so he or she understands why the price is what it is. Another example would be "Many veterinary hospitals schedule only 15-minute appointments. Your second-opinion consultation with the doctor will provide as much as 30 minutes." It's very important not to use the word "dollars." If you say the numbers but don't say "dollars," it doesn't seem as much like money to the client. (See "Five Forbidden Phrases" textbox for more caveats.)

If a caller objects to the price of a service, it's time for another value statement. A good technique is first to side with the client, so he or she feels understood, and then steer him or her to a different point of view. For example, if the caller says "This X-ray price is outrageous!" you can reply, "Yes, I can see that you might think so, because I used to think that too. But now that I've been working here and I know how much equipment and expertise are involved, I understand why that price was set." This is a way to show empathy and understanding of the client's point of view before attempting to change his or her opinion.

Don't forget to use empathy when talking to first-time callers. If the caller says he or she would like to know the price for puppy vaccinations, start with "Having a puppy in the house is so much fun! Let me tell you about our puppy-care packages."

Another tactic to use with phone shoppers is to tell them your practice's unique selling points. What makes you different? Every clinic can give a series of puppy vaccinations. Maybe yours also takes the time to "teach you everything you need to know to have a healthy, happy dog, whether you've had many dogs before or this is your first one." "We make sure you are informed about new treatments and improvements in veterinary care every time you come in for a routine exam."

SCRIPTS FOR HANDLING PHONE-SHOPPER QUESTIONS

Think about and practice what you will say in response to common client questions. As a team, you'll want to discuss your practice's selling points and come up with the best scripts, and then teach them to each new team member. For example, if a caller asks, "How much do you charge for a distemper shot for a dog?" you might answer, "Well, our prices may actually be higher than some of our competition, because we spend more time with you at each appointment and allow plenty of time for questions. We feel that we have the best veterinarians around and we will give your pet excellent, up-to-date care. But let me answer your question: Is this a puppy or an adult dog?"

If they say it is a puppy, ask, "How old is your puppy?" Let's say the client says the puppy is eight weeks old. You could say, "Oh, that's a cute age. What do you call him?" The client answers that it is Barney. Here is a sample script for the response:

> Well, Barney is at just the right age to start on one of our puppy packages. We have two packages, each of which covers all the routine vaccinations and stool checks that Barney will need. The higher-level package also includes Lyme disease vaccinations if Barney would have a risk for that disease. The doctor can discuss which package is best for you when you

---

FIVE FORBIDDEN PHRASES

Sometimes, costly business mistakes can happen in only four to six seconds after picking up the phone. Here are five forbidden phrases. Don't use these when talking to a customer:

1. **"I don't know."**

   There is no need ever to utter these words. If you don't know, find out. Instead, say, "Gee, that's a good question. Let me check and find out."

2. **"We can't do that."**

   This one is guaranteed to get your customer's blood boiling. Instead, say, "That's a tough one. Let me see what I can do to help you."

3. **"You'll have to . . ."**

   Clients don't have to do anything except die and pay taxes. Use the phrase "You'll need to . . ." or "Here's how we can help with that . . ." or "The next time that happens, here's what you can do. . . ."

4. **"Hang on a second."**

   This one is just plain annoying. Instead, say, "It may take me two or three minutes to look that up. Are you able to hold while I check?"

5. **"No."**

   Especially at the beginning of a sentence, this word conveys total rejection. Turn every answer into a positive response instead: "We aren't able to refund your money, but we can replace the product at no charge."

come in. The price for the first visit on either package is $_____, and the packages save you about 10 percent over buying each vaccine separately. At Barney's first visit, he'll receive his first distemper vaccination, a vaccination for kennel cough, a thorough examination, a stool sample check, his first heartworm pill, and a notebook and sample kit containing veterinary care instructions and information on housetraining and socialization. Would you like to set up that first appointment now?

If the potential client says yes, set up the appointment and ask him or her to bring in a stool sample and any paperwork about the pet. (See the "Appointments" section in this book.)

If he or she says "Not yet," thank the client for calling, offer to send a brochure and information on the puppy packages, and tell him or her to please call again with any further questions.

You've assured the caller that the practice is friendly, that you know what care is needed for the pet, and that the client can save a little money by getting the package. Notice how conversational this is. People like to talk about their pets and to feel they are speaking with someone who cares. You have also given the client a lot of extra information.

If the phone shopper is calling about an adult animal, ask if he or she has recently moved to this area or is seeing another veterinarian. If the caller is considering switching clinics and will tell you why, you may be able to obtain information that will allow your hospital to avoid doing whatever the other hospital did wrong. If the shopper has moved to your area from far away, there may be vaccinations or other services his or her pet needs that it didn't need where they previously lived.

If a client calls to ask the price of a surgery, you must first find out if he or she is already a client. If so, ask for his or her name and the pet's name. Tell the caller that the surgery price is based on the health status of the pet and ask him or her to hold for a minute so you can check the file. This gives you time to pull up the file and ensure there are no problems with the pet that you should know about. For example, maybe the puppy never finished its vaccination series and needs to complete that before the surgery.

If the animal is young and current on vaccinations, go ahead and quote the surgery price, explain the length of stay in the hospital and what your price includes, and set up the appointment, if possible.

If the pet's vaccinations are not current and your hospital requires them for surgery, do not say, "We require that he be current on all shots." That sounds cold and bureaucratic. Rather, say, "For the safety of your pet and the others in the hospital, we want to make sure your pet is fully vaccinated and is free of parasites before we perform the surgery. I notice on your record that Fluffy has not completed her series of puppy shots, so we would like [not 'need,' 'request,' or 'have to'] to see Fluffy before the surgery to do that." Remember that you are promoting good health care, not rules and regulations.

> Be enthusiastic and creative.

If the caller is not already a client, start with another sales pitch. For example: "We may be a little higher or lower than other clinics in the area. We want you to know that your pet will be operated on by an experienced doctor who uses gas anesthesia because it is safer for your pet. We also use a separate sterile surgery pack for each animal, and anesthesia is monitored by a licensed technician. How old is your dog and what breed is she?"

You must be truthful here or you are liable for fraud. If your surgeon just graduated from school, don't say he or she is experienced. If you don't use gas anesthesia, don't say you do. The best way to remember what to say here is to post cue cards by the phone. Your clients can't see you reading your script over the phone, and this helps you remember your own hospital's selling points and avoid sounding tentative.

Say a few sentences and then ask a question to keep the client involved and listening. Don't go on and on for 10 minutes without stopping, or you'll lose the client's attention and focus.

After the caller has told you the age and breed of the pet, tell him or her the price. If you offer options such as pre-anesthetic blood work at the time of surgery, use the sentence "The surgery starts at $_____, which will include the anesthetic, the day's stay in the hospital, and so on." Then go on to mention the options you will offer when the pet comes in for surgery. The speech could be something like this:

The surgery starts at $270, which will include pre-anesthetic blood testing and pain medication. The pain medication is a benefit many other clinics do not offer. There may be some other options you'll want at the time of surgery, such as hip X-rays or a microchip. We'll send you information on those options before the surgery date. The surgery price does include the surgery itself, the anesthetic, IV fluids during surgery, a sterile surgery pack and prep, and the hospital stay. Would you like to set up the surgery at this time?

If the client wants to set it up, ask about the vaccine status of the pet. You might also ask about fecal exams. Again, explain that you want these things done for the sake of the pet, not because "these are the rules."

When clients do not want to set up an appointment, thank them, ask them to call if they have further questions, and offer to mail them more information. Feel free to say good things about your clinic if you think they apply. Phrases like "Oh, Dr. Martin raises that breed!" or "Our clinic is certified by the American Animal Hospital Association" or "We are proud to have won a Practice of Excellence award from a veterinary journal last year" are great. There is nothing wrong with telling people you are proud to work at your hospital and that the team members are wonderful, caring, and compassionate. If you think these things are true (and if you don't, maybe it's time to start looking for a new clinic yourself!), then all you need to do is communicate that confidence to the client. Clients want to feel proud of their pet's clinic and to go to the "best" hospital around. Toot your horn! Nobody else is going to do it for you.

> **Rehearse!**

Post the good points about your hospital right by the front-desk phones so you don't forget what to say. Team members can carry cue cards in their pockets, keep a binder handy at the front desk, or enter notes into the computer to pull up when needed. These cards have scripts you write yourself based on the scripts in this book. You will remember them better having written them on your own. You can use phrases comfortable for you that are already part of your speech patterns. These might be "I'd be happy to do that for you," "Certainly, we can set that up for you," and "Of course we can."

REMINDER CALLS

Phone scripts are also important when you are making calls for overdue vaccinations. Always introduce yourself first before you ask for the person you want to speak with. If you give your name first, the client will know you are not a solicitor and will be less likely to be rude or defensive.

If you know which person in the household has primary responsibility for the pet, ask for him or her. (Whenever you see a new client and pet, ask who has the most responsibility for the pet.) Say, "Hi, this is Ellen, from Companion Animal Hospital. Is this Ms. Smith? . . . The doctors and I noticed that FiFi was due for her annual visit last week. Is everything okay with FiFi?" If the answer is "yes," say, "Well, good. I'm calling today to set up that appointment for her."

A message left on an answering machine could say, "Hi, this is Ellen from Companion Animal Hospital. The doctors and I noticed that FiFi was due for her annual visit last week. If everything is okay with FiFi, we would like to set up an appointment for her. Please call us back at . . ."

These scripts convey caring on the part of the team member making the call. They also give the owner an opening to say, "We gave FiFi away last year" or the like.

Try not to leave messages with a child or another non-decision-maker for the pet. You can say, "Do you make the health-care decisions for FiFi or should I speak with Ms. Smith instead?"

Here is a dental reminder script: "Hi, Ms. Jones. This is Emily from Norwich Animal Care. The last time we saw Henry, the doctor talked to you about his periodontal and gum disease, and how that would affect his health. It is painful, and infection can spread in the mouth and to other important organs. I'm calling today to schedule a dental appointment. When would you like to set that up?"

When clients refuse because of lack of money, offer CareCredit or let them pay half at the time of the visit and leave a held check or credit card—or tell them about whatever payment options your clinic offers. If they still can't pay—for whatever reason—say, "We don't want Henry to be in pain. When do you think you might be able to do this? We'll check back then." Write a note on the calendar or enter a callback into your computer so you remember to call Ms. Smith at that time.

If the client doesn't say why he or she is refusing needed care, ask! Use the phrase "What is stopping you from getting this care for Henry?" or "Is there a particular reason you are hesitating?" or "Is this not the level of care you want for Henry?" Address individual issues that arise, such as fear of anesthesia: "Ms. Smith, I know it seems scary, but the risk of dental anesthesia is far lower than the risk of untreated disease. We can do blood work and an ECG ahead of time so we know Henry is healthy enough to handle the anesthetic."

Be patient and be persistent. You may not enjoy making these types of calls, but they make a big difference in the quality of life that pets can enjoy.

> Be patient and keep trying.

It may seem like a lot of effort to prepare these sales scripts. But as any telemarketer can testify, how you present your material and the words you use make a great deal of difference in your success. Even if you think your clinic is the best in the world, if you do this part of your job poorly and the client goes elsewhere, you won't get the opportunity to prove it.

RESOURCES

Smith, Carin. 2009. *Client Satisfaction Pays: Quality Service for Practice Success*, 2nd ed. Lakewood, CO: AAHA Press.

Soares, Cecilia J. 1999. *One Client at a Time: Communicating the Value of Your Services*. DVD and workbook. Lakewood, CO: AAHA Press.

URINARY DISORDERS

Some of the most common medical and behavior questions you will be asked concern urination in inappropriate places. Urinary accidents and spraying can be medical, behavioral, or both. In the case of urinary behavioral issues, this is literally a life-or-death issue for the pet and should be handled promptly and well to avoid a quick trip to the local branch of the Humane Society for the pet. With medical problems, such as urinary obstruction, the prognosis can be equally dire, requiring prompt care and treatment.

Urinary problems of all sorts are extremely common in pets. According to Veterinary Pet Insurance (VPI), lower urinary tract disease is the number one medical condition affecting cats. Chronic renal failure is second, and diabetes is fifth—both lead to one of the most common symptoms of illness, PU/PD, or polyuria polydipsia, which means the pet is urinating and drinking a lot. Bladder and kidney stones, incontinence, and submissive wetting are all common issues for dogs.

Any pet that is urinating inappropriately should have a urine sample checked and a good physical exam, often including blood testing. Vaginitis, bladder infection, Feline Lower Urinary Tract Disease (FLUTD), diabetes, liver or kidney disease, arthritis, and many other diseases must be ruled out before the problem can be addressed. You'll need to have educational materials available for all these different topics.

Many genetic diseases manifest themselves with urinary tract symptoms. Some breeds of dogs are prone to specific types of bladder stones. Urine or blood screening can be done for some of these diseases. Radiographs and ultrasound scans may be utilized in diagnosing them as well. Special diets are often used for these problems and can greatly improve life expectancy or reduce risk.

If the problem is behavioral, not medical, a good history covering when and how the behavior started is needed to formulate a treatment plan (see the "Questioning Your Clients" section). Many products are available now for treating both medical and behavioral causes of abnormal urination, such as pheromone products; antianxiety medication; and supplements, such as cranberry extracts and phenylpropanolamine. You'll need to be knowledgeable and helpful if a client is to get the benefit of using any of these.

For any unneutered pet, the solution to a housetraining problem is usually neutering. For young pets or pets already neutered, training or rehabituating them to urinate in the right place will be needed. Often it is the owner who needs training, not the pet, so make appropriate educational materials available to them.

Clients often have misconceptions about urinary problems. Careful discussion is needed to reeducate the owner in such cases. For instance, cats and dogs do not urinate on carpets out of spite. They may, however, do it instinctively when stressed or when they feel their territory is threatened. Punishing the pet for urinary accidents is rarely successful and leads to more stress for the pet; therefore, any efforts by the client to physically punish the dog or cat should be strongly discouraged.

It is important to listen to clients carefully and ask questions when serious urination or defecation problems related to behavior arise. Without some background information, you will not be able to solve the problem. You need to know when and where the dog or cat is urinating or defecating inappropriately and for how long. You also need to know whether there have been changes in the household, and for cats where the litter boxes are located, what type of litter is used, and which cleaning products have been used. It may not occur to the client that the cat isn't using the litter box because it's right next to the scary washing machine.

Two handouts that you can give to cat owners appear at the end of this section. These handouts were distributed by the Wisconsin Cat Club, now called Cats International, for prevention and treatment of litter-box avoidance in cats. You can use them whenever there is a urinary behavioral problem not caused by a physical disease. "An Ounce of Prevention . . ." is a good overview of avoiding litter-box problems in the first place and would be appropriate for any cat or kitten owner. Both handouts are available at this book's companion website, www.aahanet.org/EYC/, and can be printed on two sides of the same sheet. You can also offer to mail these to any client who calls with a question on this topic. In addition, Patricia McConnell has a great booklet on feline urinary behavior problems called *The Fastidious Feline* (see Resources).

A few cats simply seem to have peculiar litter-box preferences. Some like smooth or soft surfaces and will often use the bathtub or the floor next to the litter box. Declawed cats have a reputation for doing this more often than others. Tell clients to try offering the cat an empty litter box or one lined only with newspaper in these cases. Other cats prefer carpet, so putting a piece of carpeting next to the box or on a ledge around it may be helpful, so the cat can scratch on its favorite substrate after using the box. The texture of the surface the cat digs in after using the box is important to it. A few cats will only use dirt or sand.

Make a follow-up phone call in a few days to see if the client has questions about the advice in the handouts, and call again later to see how things are going. If you don't give up on the client, many times the client won't give up on the pet. Just knowing you are still there to help them figure out what to do will give them hope that the problem can be solved. Dealing with urinary behavior problems successfully can save the lives of many of your patients.

For dogs, training must be set up so the pet can succeed and be praised for urinating in the area the owner desires. Punishment is not appropriate, and you may need to repeat this to the owner several times and in more than one way or context. In difficult cases, especially in adult dogs, the pet should be crated or tethered to the owner on a 4- to 6-foot lead whenever it is in the house so it is never unsupervised—or allowed to fail. The more times the pet is allowed to sneak away and have an accident out of sight of the owner, the worse the problem becomes. Solving house-soiling problems is possible with patience, persistence, and a systematic plan.

Be sure the dog is taught a signal that will indicate to the owner when it has to go outside. The dog may understand it should go potty outside, but if it hasn't learned to bark or paw at the door when it has to go, there will still be accidents in the house. Hanging a bell on a ribbon by the door and helping the pet ring it with its paw every time it is taken outside quickly teaches the dog to go to the door and make a motion with its foot when it needs to go out (visit www.Poochiebells.com for bells made specifically for this purpose).

> *Solving house-soiling problems is possible with patience, persistence, and a systematic plan.*

Be sure the pet goes out the same door and to the same area of the yard every time it goes outside. When the dog urinates or defecates, it should be praised with a code phrase such as "Good dog, go potty." Eventually the pet is taught to urinate or defecate on command with this phrase.

Until potty habits are established, outdoors should be for potty time only, not for playtime or running around loose. This means the pet will learn to go potty sooner—ideally on command—instead of thinking outside is for playtime. This makes it less likely the client will be standing out in the snow or sleet, waiting for the dog to pee, while the pet goofs off, thinking outside is for fun and not business.

I certainly don't have space here to teach a course on solving behavior problems related to urination, but now you have an idea of where to start and what's involved in treating some of these problems. In most clinics, one or more doctors or team members can and should develop some expertise in behavior management so that you can refer questions on these matters to someone who can solve them.

As with most behavior problems, make sure your clients know that help is available before they give up and take the pet to the shelter. Urinary behavior problems are a primary reason for Humane Society surrenders and euthanasia.

Preventing and treating behavior problems are at least as important as medical care and treatment to lengthen and improve pets' lives.

RESOURCES

Cats International, CatsInternational.org. This website has lots of useful information, including behavior handouts for clients. Click the "Articles" tab and look for "Overcoming Stress and Housesoiling."

DVM360, www.dvm360.com. This site has a history form for house-soiling behavior. Look under the "Business Center" menu and click on "Patient Forms" to find "Help Clients Get to the Source of Housesoiling Problems." Under "Client Handouts" you'll find "10 Easy Steps to Housetrain Your Dog" and "When Your Pet Doesn't Urinate Normally."

McConnell, Patricia B. 1998. *The Fastidious Feline*, and *Way to Go! How to Housetrain a Dog of Any Age*. 2003. Black Earth, WI: Dog's Best Friend. See www.dogsbestfriendtraining.com. Dog's Best Friend also carries Dr. McConnell's booklets on other behavior problems, including separation anxiety, living with multiple dogs, leadership, and other topics. They are inexpensive resources that you can sell to clients.

Overall, Karen L. 1997. *Clinical Behavioral Medicine for Small Animals*. Oxford, UK: Mosby Year Book. This is a great textbook on behavioral medicine, with a large pull-out section of client handouts on many problem behavior topics, including inappropriate urination.

LITTER-BOX PROBLEMS CAN BE PREVENTED: "AN OUNCE OF PREVENTION…"

1. Have your cat spayed or neutered at six months of age. Sexually mature, intact cats frequently use urine and fecal marking to indicate their territory. Neutering will correct 90 percent of elimination problems.

2. The rule of thumb for the number of litter boxes is one per cat in the household, plus one. Extra litter boxes are necessary because some cats like to defecate in one and urinate in another. Others will not use a box that has already been soiled or used by another cat.

3. Clean the litter boxes DAILY. The single most common reason for a cat's refusal to use a litter box is that the box is dirty. Non-clumping litter should be scooped daily and the litter box emptied and washed every other day. Clumping litter should also be scooped daily and the litter boxes washed when soiled.

4. Choose a litter that appeals to the cat. Most cats prefer the texture of the sandlike scooping litters. Be sure to choose a brand that clumps into a firm ball, making scooping easier and cleaner.

5. NEVER use scented litter. Perfumed, chemical scents repel cats. When you wash the litter box, use a mild dishwashing liquid. Do not use harsh chemicals that will leave an odor.

6. Do not use litter-box liners—they can be irritating to some cats. Also, covered or hooded litter boxes may be offensive to some cats. Be sure the litter box is not too small for your cat. The minimum size for a litter box is 22" x 16" and some cats prefer much larger pans.

7. Place litter boxes in quiet, private places that are easily accessible to the cat and where it will not be disturbed by children or ambushed by other pets. Noisy areas near washing machines, furnaces, or under stairs may frighten the cat away from the box. A house with several stories should have a litter box on each floor. NEVER place litter boxes near food and water dishes.

8. Kittens have an innate predisposition to use loose material as their litter, but they may also choose other locations. Limit their territory until they learn that the litter box is the only acceptable place for elimination. Praise and rewards will speed up the learning process. Like small children, they should not be expected to travel very far to find their toilet areas.

9. When introducing a new cat into the home, confine the cat to one room with its litter box, bed, food, and water, until the cat has used the litter box several times and shows an interest in exploring the rest of the house.

10. Help your cat feel comfortable in its own home and territory. Play games with it, give it a massage, talk to it frequently. Give it positive and affectionate attention. A confident, secure, contented, and relaxed cat does not need to relieve anxiety and stress by such extreme measures as urine or fecal marking.

Handout courtesy of Betsy Lipscomb, Cats International, www.catsinternational.org.

WHAT TO DO IF YOUR CAT IS NOT CONSISTENTLY USING THE LITTER BOX: "... A POUND OF CURE"

1. Have your cat examined by a veterinarian for a physical problem. Be sure to mention the cat's urination and defecation habits. If a cat's elimination is painful, it may associate the litter box with pain and choose to eliminate elsewhere. When the cat is healthy again, a careful reintroduction to the box will be necessary.

2. Carefully check the 10 steps for preventing litter-box problems. Are you following all of them? Perhaps the solution is as easy as adding more litter boxes, cleaning more frequently, or changing the brand of litter. Try to accommodate kitty's preferences for location and litter material whenever possible.

3. Never punish the cat for eliminating outside of its litter box. House-soiling occurs when the litter box, its contents, or its location is offensive to the cat or when the cat is stressed by the environment. Punishment only increases the cat's stress. HOUSE-SOILING IS NEVER DONE TO SPITE THE OWNER.

4. If aversion to the litter box can be ruled out, consider that the problem could be anxiety related. Has there been a change in the household? Any intrusion on the cat's territory, whether human, animal, or even a new piece of furniture, can cause a cat to feel threatened, insecure, and stressed. This results in its need to remind itself and the world of its territory. Territorial marking is usually accomplished by spraying urine on vertical surfaces, or, less frequently, by squatting and urinating or defecating on horizontal surfaces. The more cats in the household, the more likely it is that one or more of them will spray.

5. Try to relieve or eliminate the source of the cat's anxiety. (For example, pull the drapes so that kitty cannot view the antics of the tom cat next door.) If the environmental cause that triggers the territorial behavior cannot be identified or eliminated, consult with an experienced feline behavior counselor.

6. Whatever the cause for the inappropriate elimination, a brief confinement period may be necessary in order to clean the soiled areas. Place deterrents in these spots and purchase more litter boxes or new litter. The confinement room should be a comfortable room and should contain two litter boxes, fresh food and water, a bed, and toys. (Remember not to place the litter boxes near the food and water.) Visit kitty regularly, but don't let it out until the home environment has been cleaned and the litter-box situation has been improved. (Please note that extended periods of confinement may be detrimental to the retraining process.) When kitty is let out, it is important to PRAISE APPROPRIATE BEHAVIOR.

7. To thoroughly clean the urine-soaked areas, a black light may be used to identify the problem spots and a strong enzymatic cleaner should be used to saturate and neutralize them. Products available through veterinary clinics have proven to be highly effective. To repel kitty from previously soiled areas, cover them with a vinyl carpet runner (upside down!), a solid air freshener (preferably a citrus scent), or bowls of dry cat food.

Solving house-soiling problems is possible—with patience, persistence, and a systematic plan for retraining.

Handout courtesy of Betsy Lipscomb, Cats International, www.catsinternational.org.

VACCINATIONS

Vaccinations have been a mainstay of veterinary medicine for many years and have extended the lives of millions of pets. Most clients take vaccinations for granted and are happy to let the veterinarian decide which vaccines are needed for their pets.

Unfortunately, this does not mean there is anything simple about vaccinations. There are a large number of different vaccines available for pets, a larger number of vaccine protocols, and an even larger number of opinions as to which protocols are most appropriate and why. For current vaccine guidelines from the American Animal Hospital Association, visit aahanet.org.

The veterinarian will decide which vaccines are right for pets in your area and under which circumstances they are needed. There is general agreement that distemper vaccinations are necessary for virtually every pet, although the frequency of the booster vaccinations varies from practice to practice. Distemper virus itself has been virtually eliminated among pets in most of the United States, but it remains common in feral cat populations and in areas where vaccination is not as common. In the 1990s, a small town in Alaska saw a distemper outbreak that killed almost every dog there, several hundred in all, because it had no resident veterinarian and a large population of unvaccinated dogs. Cat distemper, a much hardier virus than dog distemper, can survive for years in the environment, waiting for the next unlucky cat to come along.

Cat distemper, a much hardier virus than dog distemper, can survive for years in the environment, waiting for the next unlucky cat to come along.

Wolves, foxes, coyotes, raccoons, feral cats and dogs, and other species of wildlife carry distemper viruses and can transmit them to pets through infected droppings. Both cat and dog distemper viruses are hardy enough to be transferred to a pet via shoes or clothing—as is parvovirus. Many of the respiratory diseases of cats and dogs are airborne and can waft in through an open window. Even indoor pets are at risk and should be vaccinated regularly.

Explaining vaccinations to your clients isn't difficult because you do not need to go into a lot of detail. Most clients have no idea what most of the diseases they vaccinate their pets against are, and they don't want a course on the matter—they just want to get it done. There is usually no need to go into detail about each disease in the multivalent (combination) vaccines. If a client asks what the letters stand for in the vaccine acronym, you can certainly give them a full explanation, but usually it's quite sufficient to say it is a "six-in-one distemper" or "four-in-one distemper that also protects against three upper respiratory diseases." Nor is it usually necessary to explain why the intervals between initial vaccinations is important. You can say, "The timing between immunizations is important for Bitsy to develop good immunity. We need to see her back around May 1 for her next booster."

When clients call about a new puppy or kitten, the most important thing is to get them in for an exam so you can present many preventive care topics. This includes setting up a vaccination schedule for the pet. It's best not to wait until the next booster is due several weeks later to make the appointment because you'll lose the earliest opportunity to get that pet started on heartworm and intestinal parasite control. We also want the chance to teach the client what to do during the all-important socialization period in the pet's development. At the first visit, we'll go over behavioral and nutritional care that is crucial for a young pet. No matter what the age, if a client just got a new pet you need to schedule an exam within a few days.

Do not give puppy and kitten owners too much choice in vaccine protocols. Tell them what your clinic's standard protocol is for their pet's risk factors, and administer those vaccines unless the owner refuses them. After all, we are the experts on contagious diseases, not the client. Which vaccines your hospital recommends—and under what circumstances—will depend on the philosophy of your clinic and the prevalence of certain diseases in your area.

Your clinic may offer standardized vaccination packages for puppies and kittens. Each includes the distemper series, rabies vaccination, and two stool checks, according to regular protocols. Kitten packages should also include feline leukemia (FeLV) and feline immunodeficiency virus (FIV) testing. FeLV vaccinations can be part of your standard package or be included only in a "plus" version, depending on your hospital's protocols. Puppy packages can include one or two Bordetella vaccinations. Noncore vaccines such as Lyme disease and canine influenza may be included depending on region and protocols. About 95 percent of my clients who have puppies and kittens young enough to qualify for a package purchase one.

A special note on feline leukemia and feline immunodeficiency virus: Some 3 to 6 percent of all cats in the United States are carrying either FeLV or FIV. In cats with clinical illness, 9 to 15 percent have FeLV and 9 to 12 percent have FIV (Tilley et al. 2008). More cats die of feline leukemia than any other infectious disease, more than 1 million annually in the United States alone. FIV accounts for the deaths of 2 to 3 percent of all cats in the United States.

> ***More cats die of [FeLV] than any other infectious disease, more than 1 million annually in the United States alone. FIV accounts for the deaths of 2 to 3 percent of all cats in the United States.***

Health-care packages are like McDonald's "Happy Meals." Clients like to purchase something easy and inclusive. They also like knowing the doctor will figure everything out for them and they don't have to worry about it. They have enough to cope with in housetraining and all the other excitement that comes with getting a new pet. Packages give them a small discount. The client pays for half of the package at each of the first two visits. There are four visits in the program, so the client receives a discount in exchange for getting the payments in early in the program. While on the package, clients also save the cost of the office visit for any additional exams that would have been needed for accidents or illness.

When kittens or puppies are a little older and can start on FeLV, FIV, or Lyme disease vaccinations, if indicated, spend more time talking about the risks for these diseases and whether the vaccines are appropriate for the pet. Provide handouts on these diseases at that time. At the very last vaccination visit, discuss the importance of future annual boosters and checkups. Keep in mind that the vaccinations are only one small part of the client-education picture. Puppy and kitten visits are also your opportunity to discuss nutrition, behavior, dental care, grooming, and all the other topics important to pets' health. The vaccines are a nice hook to get clients in the door, but they are certainly not the only reason for the patient visit.

Rabies vaccinations are another mainstay of medicine. Rabies vaccination of pets has reduced the number of rabies cases in people as well as in cats and dogs. In the late 1940s, more than 5,000 cases of canine rabies were reported every year. Raccoons, skunks, bats, and foxes are the most common carriers of rabies, in descending order, but bats are more likely to transmit the disease to pets and people.

People feel safe in their homes, but wildlife is right outside the door for most of us. Cats often escape outdoors—and animals sometimes make their way in. It is not uncommon in many areas of the country for people to find a bat flying around in their home. They may get into the house in a variety of ways, usually down a chimney. Raccoons can get under the porch, skunks may wander into the garage, and there may be coyotes lurking in the backyard. If the cat is vaccinated for rabies, the cat owner does not have to worry much about possible exposure to rabies. Be sure to explain this to reinforce your recommendations to clients.

Rabies vaccination also protects both the pet owner and the pet if the cat or dog bites or scratches someone. All pets should be vaccinated against rabies regularly. According to the Centers for Disease Control and Prevention, even with current rabies vaccine programs and wildlife testing protocols, more than 22,000 people require rabies injections for exposure to the virus annually. Protecting pets against rabies protects the people who live with them.

According to the Centers for Disease Control and Prevention, even with current rabies vaccine programs and wildlife testing protocols, more than 22,000 people require rabies injections for exposure to the virus annually. Protecting pets against rabies protects the people who live with them.

Most clients will agree with your clinic's vaccine recommendations, but some will request that only the rabies vaccine be given. Or they may tell you that their cat never goes outside and doesn't need a rabies vaccine, or refuse other boosters your clinic recommends. Vaccination titers may be used in some hospitals or requested by some clients. Because many clients don't know much about viral diseases or vaccines, when you meet with this resistance you may need to explain why the different vaccinations are needed and what the risk factors are for the pet. If you believe a particular patient should receive certain vaccinations and the client isn't sure, remember the repetition rule: Most people need to hear something at least five times before they act on that information. You don't need to pound any subject into the ground—nor do you need to pressure the client, whether it's for vaccinations or anything else. You do, however, need to mention the subject multiple times. These mentions can be brief, but they should be made with confidence.

Drops in human vaccination rates in the United States have led to a resurgence in preventable diseases in people. Because they may have heard or read about vaccine side effects, many parents and pet owners perceive that the risk from vaccinations is growing, although in reality, vaccines are becoming safer.

Many people who search for information on vaccine safety do so by going online using general search engines instead of by consulting medical or official websites—or, better yet, by asking their pediatrician or veterinarian for information. Clients have a limited understanding of how vaccines work and can find a lot of misinformation when surfing the Internet (Downs et al. 2008).

Be sure that when new vaccines become available, your team takes steps to educate owners about them. As with any other product, clients won't purchase services they don't know about. The client should also be educated about any changes made in your clinic's vaccination protocol, and they should understand what side effects each vaccination could cause. Your clinic should have a handout explaining its benefits, as well as possible side effects.

Clients should also receive a written document each time the pet receives any vaccination that spells out what to watch for afterward. It should describe common side effects such as malaise and myalgia (muscle aches) and state when a side effect such as swelling, vomiting, or a lump should be reported to the veterinarian. Vaccine manufacturers often provide these free of charge or you can download one from www.dvm360.com.

As with many of the medical procedures we do every day at veterinary clinics, vaccination carries some risk, and clients need to be informed about these as well as about the benefits. Cat owners should be told about the risks for postvaccination sarcoma. Demonstrate how to check for a vaccine lump and explain when such a lump would be a concern necessitating a call to the clinic.

WHAT IS A TITER?

a titer is a lab test done to measure immune system response to an infection or vaccination. If the titer blood test for a disease, say, distemper, shows the pet has a protective titer, then the pet may not need to have a booster vaccination for distemper. Titers are not available for every disease we vaccinate against. They are expensive and they can take a couple of weeks to come back from the lab, so most hospitals don't routinely do them before vaccinating. They also only measure one component of the immune system and do not necessarily provide a complete picture.

If you cover all these bases, most of your clients will respond to your reminders and come into your office every year to update their pets' examinations and vaccinations. Remember, it's laying the groundwork early on, when the patients are puppies or kittens, that establishes the value of the annual vaccines and routine exams in clients' minds. Although many clinics have tried hard to raise the importance of the examination, many people still perceive more value in the "shots." You should promote both.

Clients new to your area or considering switching to a new clinic usually will not call you until vaccinations are due for their adult pets. When new patients come to your hospital because they are ill, don't forget to obtain vaccination information. You can take the best care of the pet in the world while it's sick, but if you forget to ask the client when the pet's next vaccinations are due or whether they are current, that pet will be susceptible to more illness later on. Calling for prior records and carefully entering reminders into your computer ensure there will be no lapse in care.

When established clients miss an annual booster, send a second reminder card or an e-mail notification. If there is still no response, then get on the phone. Why wait until the pet is seriously lapsed in its vaccine protection before trying to contact the owner? If you believe in good preventive care, don't send a mixed message by waiting months to contact the client. If you leave messages the client never returns, send a third reminder letter or e-mail message that explains the risks of losing vaccine protection and the importance of routine examinations. Don't wait very long before sending the letter out, or the urgency of the pet's need is lost.

Don't make the mistake of sending notices to clients that make it sound as if you think they are careless or ignorant. (Forgetful, yes. Ignorant, no.) Every call you make and every card, e-mail, or letter you send should convey the message that you care about the pet and are concerned for its health. A caring attitude is what clients like about a practice in the first place.

Continue that caring attitude when clients actually bring the pet in for vaccinations. Treat the pet carefully and gently. Be welcoming to the pet owners even if they waited until the vaccination was overdue. Greet them with a smile and say, "We're so glad to see you! It's so good that you are getting Fluffy's vaccinations updated today." Owners don't like to see their animals hurt or frightened, and they don't like to be made to feel guilty, either. Assume that clients are doing their best with everything that is on their plate. It's your job to make both the patient and the owner feel comfortable and cared for. That way, they'll both be back again for another vaccination next year.

RESOURCES

American Animal Hospital Association. "Canine Vaccine Guidelines Revised." http://secure.aahanet.org/eweb/dynamicpage.aspx?site=resources&webcode=CanineVaccineGuidelines.

American Association of Feline Practitioners. "2006 Feline Vaccine Advisory Panel Report." www.catvets.com/uploads/PDF/2006_Vaccination_Guidelines_JAVMA_Plus.pdf. For other links, see www.catvets.com/professionals/guidelines/publications/?Id=176.

"Communicating Your Vaccine Protocol." 2007. *Veterinary Economics*, September 1.

DVM360, www.dvm360.com. DVM360 has a "Vaccine Information Form." Under the "Business Center" menu, choose "Patient Care Forms," "Practice Forms," or "Client Handouts"; it's listed under all of them. Under "Client Handouts" you'll also find "What You Should Know About Vaccines in Your Pets."

Madsen, Laura McClain. 2008. "Talking to Clients About Vaccine Protocols." *Veterinary Economics*, January 1.

Rudolph, Liza W. 2010. "How Safe Are Your Vaccine Procedures?" *Firstline*, June. http://veterinaryteam.dvm360.com/firstline/Veterinary+team/How-safe-are-your-vaccine-procedures/ArticleStandard/Article/detail/673686.

WEIGHT CONTROL AND EXERCISE FOR PETS

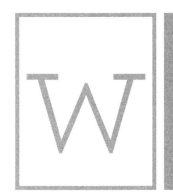

Obesity is the most common nutritional disease of pets, affecting millions of dogs and cats. According to the Association for Pet Obesity Prevention (APOP), 45 percent of dogs and 58 percent of cats are overweight or obese. Obesity is a life-shortening disease. Research has shown that the average life expectancy of an obese pet is 30 percent shorter than that of a normal-weight pet (Kealy et al. 2002; Lawler et al. 2005; Scarlett and Donaghue 1998). Excess weight is also one of the most important factors in the development of arthritis. A 10 to 15 percent weight loss results in improved clinical signs of arthritis, and a weight loss of as little as 5 to 10 percent improves mobility, according to pet owners (Impellizeri et al. 2000). Few things can improve an animal's life expectancy and quality of life more than good weight management.

> *Research has shown that the average life expectancy of an obese pet is 30 percent shorter than that of a normal-weight pet.*

Keeping weight off is a key to preserving joint health for at-risk pets. Fat cells are not inert. In fact, they produce chemicals called *adipokines* that circulate throughout the body and affect other cells. This is in part why obesity increases the risk for so many other diseases, such as diabetes, heart disease, joint disease, and urinary tract problems. It's not just the excess pounds of fat, it's the chemicals those fat cells are secreting that are so damaging (Laflamme 2007; Trayhurn 2006; Trayhurn and Wood 2005).

Fat cells produce toxins that damage other cells, leading to increased risk for cancer in dogs, cats, and humans. In some breeds, there are other health issues that arise from obesity as well. Diabetes, hepatic lipidosis, and arthritis are common problems of overweight cats.

Discussing obesity with clients can be a difficult job. They don't want to believe their pets are heavy; they enjoy rewarding their pets by giving them treats; and they are often overweight themselves. Because pets don't go to the store and buy their own food, the owners are at fault when the pet is fat, but the last thing you want to do is accuse clients of being bad pet owners and overfeeding their pals. So what do you say?

As with most things, prevention is easier than cure. Talk about exercise and nutrition early and often. Warn clients when the pet is spayed or neutered that this is the time to start watching its weight. A weight gain of up to 38 percent has been reported in spayed female dogs fed freely after spaying (McGreevy et al. 2005).

You might want to add a line to your spay and neuter release form about reducing calories after this surgery. Food intake should be regulated postoperatively to avoid excessive weight gain, and a reweigh should be done a few months after surgery to catch weight gain early.

Tell owners that it's a good idea to cut back on the amount of food they give to a pet as soon as the pet starts to get a bit pudgy. In northern states, the amount should also be decreased a bit in the winter for most pets, because they get less exercise when the weather is cold. The same goes for any change that impacts the amount of exercise a pet is getting, whether it's that the client has moved to a smaller apartment or there is a new baby in the house and the dog isn't getting walked as often. Discuss using small pieces of carrot or biscuit for treats instead of a whole one. Talk about how important exercise is for good health and for preventing behavior problems. Don't wait until the pet is 30 percent above its ideal weight to address the issue.

If the dog or cat is already overweight, you can recommend a low-calorie store food or, better yet, a prescription diet. Low-calorie store brands are usually only 10 to 15 percent lower in calories than the regular varieties—enough to slow the weight gain but not enough to reverse it. Moreover, one study found that 50 percent of the "lite," "light," and "low-calorie" diets exceeded the limits on calories per cup for low-calorie diets set by government regulations. In other words, many pet foods sold as low-calorie really aren't (Freeman and Linder 2010).

> *One study found that 50 percent of the "lite," "light," and "low calorie" diets exceeded the limits on calories per cup for low-calorie diets set by government regulations. In other words, many pet foods sold as low-calorie really aren't.*

Many clients don't know how to tell if a pet is fat. Sometimes you can tell whether a pet has put on too much weight by feeling its ribs. Many times, however, pets carry their excess weight on the hips or in the belly. One useful method that you can teach clients involves looking for a waist. If the line of the belly goes up behind the ribs when the pet is viewed from the side, or the pet gets more narrow behind the ribs when viewed from above, its weight is probably fine. If the ribs or backbone can be seen, and not just felt, the pet is too thin. If the line of the belly does not go up and/or become more narrow behind the ribs, then the pet needs to lose weight.

The next thing to tell clients is "The amount of food suggested on the bag of cat or dog food is usually very generous. Many pets need far less food than the label says. Only feed what is necessary to maintain a healthy weight. The pet will get more than enough vitamins and minerals from this amount of food, unless you are feeding a poor brand of food."

You could continue with the following:

> To lose a significant amount of weight in a reasonable amount of time, you will probably need to cut back about 30 percent of calories fed. If

you switch to a reducing diet like Hill's R/D, which has about 40 percent fewer calories than regular food, you can continue to feed your pet the same volume of food, or even a little more. If you stick with your regular food, you have to cut back by about one-third. If you choose a "lite" food, you should still cut back on the amount fed by about 20 percent, and many of these diets are actually no lower in calories than a regular food.

If you offer a therapeutic diet, tell the client exactly how much to feed the pet, how many snacks to give it, when to come back for a weight check, and what to do when the weight is lost. Make sure the client is measuring portions carefully. If you are not specific, you're fighting a losing battle. Weight control is just like every other topic in this book. It takes careful client education, repetition, reinforcement, and sometimes a fair amount of nagging. Write down the goal weight, the amount of food to feed the pet, and the date of the next recheck.

Call or e-mail the owner about once a month to reweigh the pet. Each time, remind the client how much healthier the pet will be when it is thinner and praise the client for working to get there. ("I'm so glad you are still working on the weight-loss plan. Ginger will feel so much better when she reaches her target weight!") If the pet is begging and scrounging on its diet, the client can add cooked carrots, green beans, or puffed rice to a dog's meals to fill it up without adding many calories. A baby carrot is only 3 calories. A medium Milkbone biscuit, by comparison, has 110 calories.

Cats can be as bad at begging and pleading as dogs. The owner should substitute playtime or a catnip toy for food rewards. Distracting a pet from its hunger pains with a game of "fetch" or "chase the paper wad" works for both cats and dogs and the increased exercise level helps make the diet go faster. Exercising with the pet is good for the owner, too. Going for walks, learning agility training, and even doggy dancing are great for both.

Many, if not most, pets get far less exercise than they should. Lack of exercise leads to behavior problems as well as obesity. However, the pet's exercise level should not undergo a big increase suddenly. The pet should go from sedentary to active slowly, just as a person would when beginning an exercise program. If an owner is willing to invest 10 to 15 minutes per day dragging strings around the house for the cat or playing ball with the dog, it makes the weight loss go faster, improves the bond between the owner and the pet, and increases the fitness level of the pet.

Getting cats up and moving can be a challenge. A simple way to increase a cat's exercise level is to have the client divide the cat's food into small portions and distribute them around the house, so the cat has to move from place to place to eat all of it. You can spread dog food around, too, even flinging it out into the yard. This trick is best, though, for indoor cats. Puzzle toys also work for both dogs and cats. With puzzle toys, the pet's food is placed inside a toy that has to be manipulated to get the food out, keeping the pet busy and more active. It's even possible to purchase treadmills for pets, and cats will use these if they have access to them. YouTube has videos of cats running on giant exercise wheels similar to those used by rodents in their cages. Pets like to be active if they have the chance and the encouragement.

If there are children in the household, the parents can try to enlist their help in the weight-loss project because they are usually the worst offenders when it comes to giving treats to pets. You can initiate this by explaining to the child why Ginger needs to lose weight: "If she gets too fat, she could get very sick." Explain the information at the child's level. For example "One of these treats for your little dog is like a whole bowl of ice cream for you or me."

If a pet already has arthritis, diabetes, heart disease, or one of the other many problems that obesity contributes to, the weight-loss program can be set up as part of the medical treatment: "You will need to give this medication and feed this amount of this food until we see Ginger again next time."

For pets that are too thin, the answer may be as simple as increasing the amount of food the pet is fed or switching to a higher-calorie food. Any pets that are losing weight unexpectedly should have a thorough exam and blood testing. Diabetes, kidney disease, liver disease, thyroid abnormalities, heart disease, and cancer are some of the many problems that can cause weight loss. If the pet is young and active and already eating a healthy diet, the owner can add fat, such as vegetable oil, to the food to add calories. Neutering can also be helpful for overly thin pets.

Although weight gain or loss is sometimes a symptom of an underlying medical condition that requires a veterinarian's attention, many times it simply is the result of an owner's lack of knowledge as to what a healthy pet looks like, how much food the pet needs, and what type of food to feed. Helping your clients understand these things, without sounding patronizing, will extend the life span and improve the quality of life of many of your patients. If their pets are successfully nursed through a weight-loss program, owners are delighted with their increased vitality—and grateful to the veterinary team for making it possible for them to succeed.

RESOURCES

American Veterinary Medical Association. "AVMA Collections: Obesity in Dogs." www.avma.org/avmacollections/obesity_dogs/default.asp. This web page lists a collection of more than 20 articles from the *Journal of the American Veterinary Medical Association* pertaining to this topic.

Association for Pet Obesity Prevention (APOP), www.PetObesityPrevention.com.

Becker, Marty, and Robert Kushner. 2006. *Fitness Unleashed: A Dog and Owner's Guide to Losing Weight and Gaining Health Together*. New York: Three Rivers Press.

DVM360, www.dvm360.com. DVM360 has several handouts and forms on obesity-related topics. From the "Business Center" menu, choose "Client Handouts." Titles include "Pet Obesity Handout," "Pet Obesity," "Weight, Calories and Your Pet," "Teach Clients About Canine Weight Loss," "Teach Clients About Feline Weight Loss," and dog and cat "Weight Check-In Forms."

"The Finances of Fitness." 2008. *Veterinary Economics*, October 1.

"Give the Skinny on Fat Pets." 2009. *Veterinary Economics*, April 1.

PetFit.com. This website, developed by Hill's Pet Nutrition, has feeding tips, dog and cat workout tips, a weight tracker, and more.

Pet Obesity Prevention, www.petobesityprevention.com/images/calorie_treats.pdf.

X-RAYS, ULTRASOUND, AND OTHER HIGH-TECH PROCEDURES

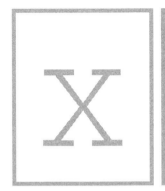

Here's the one word to remember when it comes to high-tech equipment: brag. Clients are amazed and impressed by the things veterinarians accomplish in hospitals today. Tell them about your equipment and how it could benefit their pet. Point it out on hospital tours. Demonstrate your pulse oximeter or digital radiology equipment at an open house or during Girl Scout and Boy Scout tours. Show the client a radiograph and point out the disease you see. Videotape the ultrasonic scan, put a dental X-ray in the patient record, or send home an ECG strip, test result printout, or extracted tooth. All these things lend value to pet diagnosis and treatment.

Have a speech memorized for new clients (see sample speech below). It's amazing how many clients ask, "Do you do surgery here?" or "I didn't know you had boarding!" Many clients will never read your clinic brochure, so you need to tell them and show them what you can do for them. You can also give out your business cards so that clients can call and ask for someone they know personally if they have questions later. This is especially important for large clinics with many employees because it helps clients feel a more personal bond with the practice.

Sometimes all the new technologies and practices at veterinary clinics take clients by surprise, especially if they are older and remember a simpler time when there weren't so many options. In those cases, you may want to take a different approach. One way is to use a handout like the one supplied at the end of this section entitled "Explaining Choices and the Cost of Modern Veterinary Care." This handout sympathizes with the client's view while explaining why the options and new procedures are necessary.

Below is a sample speech to use with new clients. Giving this warm, open, and welcoming speech helps clients feel knowledgeable and at home from the first visit. It can also be used for tours given to community groups or for an open house or other special occasion. Adapt it for your hospital to tell clients about all the wonderful things you offer.

> Hi, I'm Janie, and I'm a veterinary assistant here at Grafton Animal Hospital. I'd like to welcome you to our clinic and tell you a little more about it while you're waiting for the doctor.
>
> We are a full-service clinic. This means we do surgery, dentistry, X-rays, and nutritional and behavioral counseling, as well as treating sick animals and providing routine care such as vaccinations. We treat dogs, cats, birds, ferrets, rabbits, and pocket pets such as gerbils and hamsters. We also have boarding facilities, so your pet can stay here while you're on vacation.
>
> Our doctors have lots of experience and they really care about their patients. We hope you like all of them, but if you like a particular doctor better, you can request to see that doctor as long as he or she is working that day and it's not an emergency.
>
> Our goal is to give your pet excellent care and to give you excellent service. We emphasize preventive medicine to keep your pet healthy and happy as long as possible. We try to design a care program that's appropriate to your situation and your pocketbook. In other words, a hunting dog that is out in the field working hard and is exposed to ticks and other wildlife may need different nutrition and vaccinations than a poodle that lives in the house. [For cat owners, substitute the examples of an outdoor cat that hunts for mice and an indoor cat.] We believe strongly in client education. We'll teach you as much as you want to know about the health-care needs of your pet. Sometimes it may seem like we are bombarding you with a lot of information, but we want to be

sure you know about every service or product that could help your pet lead a longer, healthier life. Then we'll try to help you decide which ones are right for you and your pet.

We are very proud of our equipment and facility. We'd love for you to see them. [If there is time to tour the clinic at that point, do so.] The doctor will be in to see you shortly. Do you have any questions I can answer at this time about the hospital or our services?

With a quick 10-minute tour, you can promote just about every aspect of good care to a new client. Here is a sample of pointing out more good things about your clinic during the tour itself:

You've already seen the waiting room and exam room. Each exam room is a little bit different. Each room has a computer, so you can watch multimedia presentations on different aspects of pet care, such as dentistry or parasite prevention. Each one contains an otoscope and ophthalmoscope for examining ears and eyes, a stethoscope, and equipment for drawing blood samples or doing simple lab procedures such as skin scrapes or ear swabs to look for mites. This next exam room has a small scale for weighing birds and pocket pets and special equipment for bird care.

This area is called the pharmacy. We keep a large variety of medications in these cabinets, everything from antibiotics to medications for heart disease, urinary tract problems, ear infections, parasites, and so on. The pharmacy is also a work area for our team members.

Our medical records are all electronic. Our computers use a system designed for veterinary hospitals. Like most businesses, we'd be lost without it. The computer also stores a variety of handouts on various diseases, and we also have file drawers full of information. We try to teach clients about good pet care and also make sure you understand your pet's diseases or problems so you can help us make treatment decisions. We rarely let you leave here without reading material about your pet!

At the other end of the hall is the laboratory. We have a microscope for examining blood smears, stool samples, swabs, and the like. We have centrifuges for spinning blood and urine samples, and we have machines that allow us to analyze many different parameters, especially blood serum, for things like blood sugar or liver enzymes. We can often diagnose your pet's condition right here in the hospital. We also use this equipment every day for pre-anesthetic blood testing, to make sure your pet is healthy enough for surgery.

We also send samples out to different laboratories for other, more specialized testing. Things like tumor biopsies are sent out. For many tests, we have results back within a day.

This room holds our X-ray, or radiograph, machine. This lets us diagnose everything from a broken leg to pneumonia. Some radiographs can be taken while the animal is awake. At other times, anesthesia is needed to properly position the patient for the X-ray.

This area is for hospitalized cats. We keep them separate from the dogs so they aren't scared by the barking. Our dog ward has both runs and cages, and we can give baths here as well. We feed [brand] to our hospitalized or boarding patients if pet owners don't bring their own food along with them.

This area is the treatment room. It actually has many functions. Seriously ill animals stay next door in ICU so we can watch them closely. If your pet comes in after being hit by a car, we will bring it straight to this room for IV fluids and other emergency care. Emergency drugs and equipment are kept here. This cart contains our ECG machine.

We do dentistry in this area, using the same sort of equipment used in human dentistry. We also take full-mouth dental radiographs just as your own dentist would do. Root canals, crowns, and other advanced procedures are done on pets as well as people.

This area, called pack/prep, has our ultrasonic instrument cleaner and the autoclave, which sterilizes instruments once they are clean.

We prep surgery patients over in this area. The pet is anesthetized here and then moved to the surgery room. Along with spays, neuters, and other routine surgeries, we do all kinds of other soft-tissue and orthopedic surgeries.

This is the surgery room. We use gas anesthetic for most procedures because it is very safe. The surgery table and lights can be adjusted for different sizes of animals and different procedures. The orange pad keeps pets from getting cold during surgery. The most important piece of equipment here is the anesthetic monitoring system, which includes a pulse oximeter. It measures the heart rate and blood oxygen level of our patients under anesthesia, so we know right away if they are having any difficulties during surgery. [Here you can pause and demonstrate the pulse oximeter on a client's finger or run a recording of a previous patient—equipment is more impressive if it's running.] Next to it is our blood pressure machine, which is also used in surgery, as well as for monitoring patients with high blood pressure.

From here, we'll go back up to the exam room. The doctor is probably ready to see you now.

With this quick 10-minute tour, you've managed to promote just about every aspect of good care to the new client. Depending on what equipment you have, you can talk about lasers, ultrasound, endoscopy, rehabilitation, or any other services you want to promote. The more clients you let tour the clinic, the more clients there will be out in the community telling their friends and neighbors about all the high-tech equipment you showed them and how friendly and helpful you were. Be sure you've checked the condition of the clinic before you take clients through—if the technicians are wrestling with a nasty cat or someone just made a mess on the floor, save the tour for next time!

I'm a big advocate of cross-training the team. Everyone from the doctor to the kennel worker should know what equipment your hospital has, why it's important to patient care, and how it's used. You can also put colored stickers on important pieces of equipment so that tour guides remember to cover them all. Keep a few ear-mite or ringworm slides around to pop on the microscope for clients to view. You won't always have time for a long production; sometimes the tour may need to be shortened. But when you do have time, a tour is a great way to impress new and old clients alike. When you invite youth groups such as Scouts or elementary school groups, you will have parent chaperones in the group as well who could become future clients. In addition, you may inspire a young person to become a veterinarian or a member of a veterinary team one day.

The more equipment you have, the more items you should promote. Mention new acquisitions in a newsletter, set up a display of ultrasound scans or ECG strips in the waiting room, or give clients a copy of a computerized report. As with everything else, the more clients see or hear about a test or procedure, the more likely they are to let you use it on their own pets. So spread the word! Your hospital is the place to go for high-quality care!

EXPLAINING CHOICES AND THE COST OF MODERN VETERINARY CARE

If you are like many of our clients, you are sometimes frustrated or overwhelmed with too many choices when you visit your veterinarian. You need to choose which vaccinations your pet will receive, what flea or heartworm preventives you will use, and what tests you want your pet to undergo, whether for wellness screening or because your pet is ill. Before surgery is performed you may be asked whether you want a pre-anesthetic ECG, a nail trim, a microchip, or laser surgery. As medicine gets more complicated and more choices become available, the discomfort about all these options is only going to get worse.

As more technology becomes available, not only do we have more choices but the standard of care becomes increasingly complicated. For example, it is now the standard of care for patients to have pre-anesthetic testing and to be on IV fluids during procedures. If your pet dies under anesthesia and these services were not provided, the veterinary hospital is now liable. Every year the bar gets a little higher and the world of veterinary medicine gets a bit more complex—and costly.

You have the legal right to understand all the options available to you and to know the benefits and drawbacks of each one. Although these new standards protect you and your pet, they have their drawbacks for both you and us. Doing a surgery admission can be a bit of a hassle now, for example. We used to allow 10 minutes for that appointment but it's now 20 or more.

The cost of all these options can become overwhelming, too. Most people cannot afford to do absolutely everything that might be of benefit to their pets. The emotions we see when all these options are presented range from anger and dismay to guilt or embarrassment over not being able to afford everything available or perhaps not even wanting all these services.

It is never our intent to pressure anyone into doing anything, but it sure can make both us and you uncomfortable. Negotiating over a beloved family pet in a tight economy is not at all the same as deciding whether you want fries with your Big Mac. It's stressful and often emotional, and has the added risk that you sometimes will need to divulge personal financial information. I'm sure you often feel that we are judging you as "pet parents" based on the decisions you make, though this is never our intent. We have budgets and car repairs and kids needing braces, too. We don't expect every client to do every test or treatment, and we know that we will usually have to help you pick and choose.

When it comes to making decisions, our clients fall into three groups. Some people want us to tell them exactly what they should do. Their question is usually "What would you do if it were your pet?" Other people want us to give them information but want to make the decisions themselves. (Unfortunately, some clients want to make the decisions without listening to the options. Legally, this isn't really possible anymore because we are required to explain all the options, whether a client wants to hear them or not.) The third group of clients wants to collaborate—to discuss the options and decide together.

Having these discussions about options can be tricky. We don't always know what your preferred decision-making style is—or a husband and wife may have completely different styles or needs. We may not know whether you are one of those people who wants to do absolutely everything for their pet or one who wants only the minimum. We may not have had enough interaction with a client to build trust and rapport, which may make a client more hesitant or less trusting when decisions need to be made. In an emergency, a pet owner may be forced to make very difficult decisions rapidly without even having met the veterinarian before.

As the world becomes increasingly complicated and confusing, it's useful to keep in mind that the choices we are making today are about services and procedures that we didn't used to have available. Our typical patient lives twice as long as pets did in the 1960s because of advances in vaccines, medications, anesthesia, nutrition, and parasite control. All this new information we are throwing at you means that your pets have the opportunity to lead longer, healthier lives than ever before. It's a wonderful world of possibility, a chance to learn more about your pets and to be able to provide them with care that was unavailable just a generation ago. For a household pet these days, life is good!

YEARLY EXAMS AND SENIOR HEALTH-CARE RECOMMENDATIONS

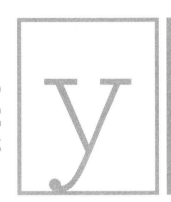

The annual or semiannual examination and vaccinations our patients receive are golden opportunities. For many clients and pets, the 15 to 30 minutes the clinical staff spend with them for their annual checkups may be the only time spent with them all year. There is only that short period of time for the doctor to examine the pet, chat with the owner, go over any problems identified, and educate the client on anything new.

From the time a client obtains a new puppy or kitten to the time the pet grows old, dozens of new products and services will be introduced that could help that pet. It's your job to explain the products or services to the clients, and you have just a few minutes a year—or four to five hours over the pet's lifetime—to do it. You need to talk about nutrition, behavior, dental care, vaccinations, skin and ear care, and flea control, among other subjects.

Do not let the few precious minutes you have with each client go to waste. Be sure you are educating them about new services and reviewing things they will need later on, and use handouts and other written materials to cover things you don't have time to go over in detail. Most of all, this is the time to ask the client lots of questions and work together to develop a health plan that's right for the pet and the family.

Senior pets should get special treatment at their yearly or twice yearly exams. I like the phrase "Senior care begins at birth." The concept of senior care beginning at birth, or even at conception, hinges on the idea of wellness care—doing the best you can throughout a pet's life to lay the foundation for the longest, healthiest life possible. It means spending time educating clients about nutrition, weight control, dental care, spaying and neutering, and all the other components of health care that influence longevity.

Senior care begins at conception because the pet's life span and disease risk are influenced by genetics, the nutrition of its mother, the breed of pet, and many other factors. We can influence many of the factors early on by teaching the client what to do, what not to do, and when to call us with a question or problem. For example, 40 percent of purebred dogs have genetic defects. Prepurchase counseling on how to shop for a healthy puppy can save pet owners thousands of dollars and a lot of heartbreak. Breed tendencies, puppy mills, temperament testing, screening tests—the list goes on. For cat owners, screenings for feline immunodeficiency virus (FIV) and feline infectious peritonitis (FIP) are important.

Our brains are programmed to respond to acute danger better than they are to plan ahead, whether it's developing a plan for hurricanes, famine, global warming, or a wellness care program. We are immersed in our hectic, busy lives and practices, and we don't usually spend enough time thinking about our missions, visions, or values—or what is really the most effective way to deliver high-quality care. For a doctor or technician, it's usually more fun and exciting to perform surgery or treat sick pets than to endlessly teach owners about preventive and wellness care. However, patients can be helped far more effectively when diseases are diagnosed and treated in their early stages than when preventive care is given short shrift.

As pets age, we should spend an increasing amount of time focusing on senior programs and common old-age diseases and problems. The veterinarian needs to develop a program and decide which tests to offer as well as when to offer them. There is little agreement as to when a pet turns "senior," what care should be instituted at what age, and what tests are most valuable.

Here are some questions that veterinarians need to answer and share with the practice team: At what age do you consider a pet senior? What care recommendations do you make for senior pets that are different from what you recommend for younger adult pets? Should you do annual blood testing starting at age nine and do it twice annually after age 12? Do you offer UPC or urine screening? BP? T4? Chest X-rays? ECG? When and why? Or if not, why not?

There isn't a right and a wrong answer for some of these questions, but all team members should be clear on what your clinic's philosophy is and why. What would team members do for their own pets? For most clients, it's a matter of how to prioritize and do what is within their budget. Your team can discuss these issues, figure out what you want to improve or measure, and then implement changes.

What diseases are commonly seen in senior pets at your clinic? What will protocols be when a problem is diagnosed? It's not enough to just gather information; you need to utilize it to improve the health of the pet. Protocols should not just be about drugs. Treating diseases in senior pets may involve nutrition, weight management, supplements, oncology, exercise and physical therapy, environmental accommodations, or education and support.

We need to teach clients carefully and thoroughly about wellness care for their older pets. Intensive monitoring of patients decreases the risk of a poor outcome, whether it's in pets under anesthesia or in emergency and critical care, in pets with chronic disease or in apparently healthy pets. A chance to diagnose disease early means a chance to intervene early. Early detection leads to better outcomes. Organ damage precedes organ failure and thus clinical signs of disease, in many cases. The clinic should emphasize wellness care with clients because it is so much better and more effective than waiting until the pet is ill and the organs have already begun to fail.

Older pets can appear healthy but still have underlying problems that can be detected when a clinic emphasizes good senior pet care. Here are some statistics: Eighteen percent of middle-aged and older cats (above age seven) that appear healthy upon physical examination have an underlying disease. Ten percent of cats over age nine have an elevated T4 level, and above age 12 that increases to 20 percent. (That's a lot of hyperthyroid cats!) Two-thirds of those cats with hyperthyroidism and/or chronic kidney disease have or will develop hypertension, and many have periodontal disease, pancreatitis, diabetes, or other health problems that need diagnosis and treatment. For senior dogs, the percentages are just as bad or worse. Twenty-three percent of senior dogs that appear healthy upon physical examination have an underlying disease. Even 5 percent of young pets that appear healthy upon physical examination have an underlying disease, and 7 percent of dogs less than eight years old have low thyroid levels (Aucoin 2006; Lund et al. 1999).

Wellness testing is not just about blood work. Other tests that may be useful are urinalysis, proteinuria/microalbuminuria, ECG screening, triponin and levels of other enzymes, X-rays, ultrasound, blood pressure monitoring, fecal testing, IOP (intraocular pressure to check for glaucoma), and STT (Schirmer tear test, to check for dry eye) monitoring—it's amazing how many problems we can catch when we start looking for them.

The whole team needs to be on board with such programs. Some team members may feel that when programs are presented in a marketing context, the programs are not about patient care but about generating income for the practice. It's important for the team to understand the benefits of senior care for the patients. Another thing that trips practice teams up is that it's easy to get bogged down in the logistics of a program and give up after the first attempt is difficult or produces inconsistent results. This is why most veterinary hospitals still are not doing much wellness testing, despite the obvious benefits to the patients.

Remember that it's not enough to recommend something, you have to teach it, repeat it, and reinforce it! Wellness programs are a lot of work. They include program development, fee setting, team training, client education, marketing, and, last, protocols. Actually implementing a program is a big hill to climb—it's complicated and time-consuming. In addition, there may be resistance to change among team members, and it's very easy to slip back into old habits and ways.

The good news is, you already have protocols in your hospital, but they probably aren't written down. Doctors use the same anesthetics, do the same physical exams, and do their spay surgeries the same way every time. Senior programs are a great place to start putting more formal protocols in place. Clarify the simple things, and add them to a binder a few at a time. Also refer to the information about establishing protocols in the "Risk Management" section of this book for more information on what to cover and how to cover it consistently and well.

Be realistic if you are just starting out planning a wellness program. Although many clients will comply, many will not. Don't get discouraged. Set goals, but don't expect 100 percent. Also, do not judge your clients! It's your role to make the recommendations. It's the pet owner's job to make the decisions. Be flexible with payment methods, with medication administration methods, and with the ways you contact the client or follow up. Offer options and let the client decide.

For many teams, getting everybody on board can be a challenge. Whenever a new program is introduced, a small percentage of team members usually support it right away and a larger percentage are automatically against it. Half the team will sit on the fence and wait to see who wins. If you plan how you will introduce a new program, it's often possible to improve these odds. Getting cooperation from team members is a lot like getting compliance from your clients. How do you do it? The same way you get client compliance!

Here are five steps to follow in team interactions when making these changes. Anyone on the practice team is in a position to influence the way the rest of the team responds. Stay positive and make sure everyone feels like a part of things.

Step 1. Explain what you want to see happen: You can say, for example, "We want all our patients to have access to the very best care."

Step 2. Explain how the change will benefit people: Use a value statement. For example, say: "Early detection of problems allows for better and more effective treatment. Senior-care programs are proven to improve quality of life and allow clients to keep their beloved older companions longer." Remind team members that all of you work in a veterinary hospital because you care about pets and people. Make sure they understand the benefits of developing new protocols for the patients and the clients.

Step 3. Discuss costs, risks, and benefits: Team members need to know specific benefits of each new protocol for pet health care. Explain why different aspects of the program will allow the clinic to take better care of its patients. Make it positive and motivate team members to strive for a goal. Perhaps you can celebrate with a party when different milestones are met. Show appreciation for all of the team's hard work: "We really appreciate those of you who have worked so hard on this project."

Step 4. Listen for feedback and address questions and concerns: Check in with team members: "Are we all in agreement that this is what we will recommend?"

Step 5. Close the sale: Team members aren't buying anything, but the sense of concluding different stages of a process is still helpful. You can say, for example, "I know that working as a team we can help a lot more senior pets."

Team meetings, leadership, and good communication skills are essential if veterinary hospital employees are ever to make improvements and work together effectively.

SENIOR CAT CARE

Old age is not a disease, it is a stage of life. None of us would be very happy with our physicians if we went to their office complaining about an ache or pain, lump or bump, and were told, "You are just getting old, and there's nothing we can do about that." Cats are often the neglected species. Their owners bring them to us less frequently than dog owners bring in their dogs, and they spend less money on their care. We often are complicit in this and don't take the time to educate cat owners as we would dog owners. There's a lot that we can teach clients about senior cat care, because they usually know very little about it.

Older cats typically spend less time grooming than younger cats do. Also, the skin and hair coat tend to become drier with age. Owners should brush mature cats frequently, thus helping to remove debris and improve the distribution of natural oils on the skin and in the hair coat. If necessary, the cat can be bathed with mild hypoallergenic, nondrying shampoo. Long-haired cats may have more problems with hair mats as they age, and the hair coat may need to be clipped to make it easier for the owner to groom the cat. Obesity and arthritis also restrict mobility and the ability to groom adequately (obese cats are five times more likely to have arthritis, and overweight cats are three times more likely to have arthritis).

Osteoarthritis is generally less severe in cats than in dogs because of the cat's light weight. Eventually, though, almost all elderly cats will become stiff and sore. There are lots of medications and treatments available for feline arthritis nowadays. Teach your clients how to recognize pain and what can be done about it.

Oral cavity disorders (periodontitis, gingivitis, stomatitis, dental disease, oral ulcers, and oral cavity tumors) are often overlooked as the cause of significant illness in older cats. Common clinical signs of oral disease are poor appetite, weight loss, halitosis (bad breath), chattering teeth, abnormal chewing and/or swallowing behavior, decreased grooming, and nasal discharge. Infection often accompanies oral cavity disease and may result in intermittent bacteremia or septicemia (bacteria entering the bloodstream or affecting the entire body). This may, in turn, lead to disorders in other body systems, including kidney, hepatitis, and possibly cardiovascular disease.

Apparent senility occurs in cats as well as dogs. Behavior changes include confusion, aimless wandering around the house, and getting trapped in a corner or under a piece of furniture. Other changes may be aggression and changes in elimination behavior. The clinic should perform a thorough examination and workup before assuming that these changes are due to senile dementia, however, because other diseases can cause similar symptoms. Impaired *thermoregulation* (ability to regulate body temperature) is another central nervous system change that may occur in older cats. Clients should be instructed to provide a safe heat source for aging cats to use as needed.

Energy requirements do not decrease in older cats. In fact, many cats absorb food from their digestive tracts less efficiently as they age. They may actually need to eat more than they used to in order to maintain their body weight. The addition of extra fatty acids, antioxidants, and fiber to an older cat's diet has been shown to extend life expectancy by over a year, and the cats that received these extra nutrients also had better quality of life and maintained their weight better in their last year of life than older

CONTINUED

CONTINUED

cats in a control group (Cupp et al. 2008). Starting an enriched diet early in life is one of the best ways you can help a cat to live longer.

The best diet for older feline patients is one that is well balanced, nutritionally complete, highly palatable, highly digestible, and replete with potassium and taurine. If the cat has a specific medical problem, such as kidney disease, that may be helped by another special diet, then that diet is the best thing to feed it—luckily, renal diets for kidney disease share many of these same properties (Rawlings et al. 2000; Planting et al. 2005).

Older cats tend to eat more meals than younger cats, but those meals tend to be smaller. Leaving food out all day may help these cats maintain good body weight. Other considerations are that some cats are social eaters (owner must be present at mealtime); prefer to eat from a flat dish or saucer rather than a small bowl, possibly because they do not like to place their face into a bowl; or have decreased saliva production that makes food taste strange or feel different than it used to.

In summary, there is much that we can do to keep our older feline friends healthy and happy. Most indoor cats that receive veterinary care throughout their lives live to be at least 15 years old, and many reach their late teens or early twenties. A little testing and a little tender loving care should keep a cat purring for a long, long time.

RESOURCES

Boss, Nan. 2003. *The Client Education Notebook: Customized Client Education Materials to Use in Your Own Practice.* Lincoln, NE: AVLS-PetCom.

DVM360, www.dvm360.com. DVM360's website has several handouts and forms on wellness visits and senior care. Under the "Business Center" menu, under "Patient Care Forms," you'll find "A Lifetime of Canine Wellness" (which also appears on the "Client Handouts" list), "Canine Annual Examination Report," and "Senior Wellness Report Card." Under "Client Handouts" you'll find "Wellness for the Older Pet," "What Is a Wellness Screen?" "A Lifetime of Feline Wellness," "Sample Senior Wellness Letter" (which also appears on the "Practice Operations Forms" list), "How Wellness Care Saves Money," "Veterinary Wellness Exam Checklist," "Pet Wellness Report Card," and a "Step by Step Guide to Talking to Clients About Wellness Programs." You can also print out flyers on junior and senior wellness testing.

Jevring, Caroline, and Tom Catanzaro. 1999. *Healthcare of the Well Pet*. Philadelphia: W. B. Saunders.

McLain, Laura. 2008. "Streamline Your Senior Care to Improve Compliance." *Veterinary Economics*, September 1.

Rothstein, Jeff. 2009. "Help Senior Pets Graduate to Good Health." *Veterinary Economics*, May 1.

ZOONOTIC DISEASES

Part of your job is to educate clients about diseases they can get from their pets, and vice versa. Sometimes this feels very awkward. You don't want to imply that having pets is dangerous or unsanitary or that people and pets can't live together safely. The idea to get across to clients is simple: "Keeping your pet safe and healthy helps protect your human family, too." This can become a mantra that you memorize and say again and again when addressing this issue with clients.

The list of zoonotic diseases transmissible from pets to humans is long. Sixty percent of the nearly 1,500 diseases recognized in people have zoonotic potential. Nearly 75 percent of newly emerging diseases, such as the Ebola virus, avian influenza, and West Nile virus, are zoonotic. Some of the more common problems—such as roundworms, fleas, sarcoptic mites, and rabies—have been briefly discussed in previous sections.

It is important to know about the dozen or so common diseases that your patients and clients can transmit to each other and to be honest with clients when discussing any of these diseases with them. If someone becomes ill with the disease his or her pet had, your clinic and doctors are liable if you haven't warned the client of the risk of transmission from the pet to the members of the family it lives with. It is also very important to know what these diseases are so you can protect yourself and other team members when handling the pets in the clinic.

Any disease showing progressive neurological symptoms, including weakness, lameness, paralysis, changes in behavior or temperament, seizures, tremors, or inability to swallow, has the potential to be rabies. Only the minimum number of people necessary should handle or treat an animal suspected of carrying rabies. Be sure your clinic has information on rabies quarantine requirements and rabies vaccine laws for your state or province, as laws and procedural requirements vary. In general, if a pet or wild animal dies with any of these symptoms, and humans or other pets may have been exposed to this animal, the animal's brain should be tested for rabies. If testing is not possible because the animal was not in good enough condition for testing, or could not be caught, the people exposed should be vaccinated against rabies.

If an animal or pet has bitten someone but has no disease symptoms, the animal must be quarantined for at least 10 days. If the animal dies while still within the quarantine period, it, too, should be tested for rabies. These precautions are taken even if the animal has a current rabies vaccination, because no vaccine is considered 100 percent effective. If a person does contract rabies, there is no cure once symptoms have begun. The disease is almost invariably fatal.

All of these facts are depressing but vital for you to know so that you can advise clients who call with questions about rabies. Again, be sure you know the exact procedures to recommend, and don't hesitate to ask a doctor to speak to the client when the subject of rabies comes up.

Intestinal parasites are big in the zoonotic hit parade as well. Roundworms, hookworms, Giardia, and toxoplasmosis all can affect humans as well as pets. When hookworm eggs are shed with a pet's stool, for example, they hatch into larvae. These larvae get into the next pet or person by burrowing into the skin, usually on the feet. They can cause a severe, ugly rash in humans. Roundworm eggs survive for years in the soil and can cause gastrointestinal and neurological disease.

The important thing to remember is the simple advice to "wash your hands," and if you've been out in your yard barefoot, wash your feet as well. Parents should be aware of these parasites because children playing in gardens, sandboxes, and litter boxes are especially at risk. Wash your own hands thoroughly in soap and warm water after handling all stool specimens, and advise your clients and coworkers to do the same. Pregnant women should avoid cleaning litter boxes during the first trimester of pregnancy and should wear plastic or rubber gloves if they must do this chore.

> **When hookworm eggs are shed with a pet's stool, they hatch into larvae. These larvae get into the next pet or person by burrowing into the skin, usually on the feet. They can cause a severe, ugly rash in humans.**

You may get calls from pregnant clients whose physicians recommend blood testing of household cats for toxoplasmosis. Unfortunately, the test tells you if a cat has been exposed to toxoplasmosis but not whether it is shedding the parasite in the stool. I always advise my clients who are pregnant that regardless of the test results, they should not be the ones cleaning the box! This is a good way for a pregnant woman's partner or a friend or relative to pitch in and help during the pregnancy.

Bacterial infections such as salmonella and *E. coli* can also be acquired via fecal material, as can the protozoan Cryptosporidium. These are other good reasons to be careful handling diagnostic testing of animal feces. Animals eating raw and homemade diets are more likely to be shedding these forms of bacteria, which is why pets on raw diets are typically not accepted for hospital or nursing-home visitation programs.

Another type of bacterial infection that is of zoonotic concern is MRSA. The acronym stands for "methicillin-resistant *Staphylococcus aureus*," and it refers to typically human staph infections that are resistant to antibiotics. Dogs usually harbor and become infected with *Staphylococcus intermedius* instead of *S. aureus*, but cases of MRSA have been reported in animals, and animals can also become carriers of this type of infection. Since MRSA has been moving from hospitals into communities, we will be hearing more about the zoonotic potential of these bacteria in the future.

Other bacterial infections that can be transmitted to people from pets—or vice versa—are Streptococcus bacteria, which cause strep throat; Bartonella, which causes "cat scratch fever"; and Leptospirosis, which causes severe liver or kidney disease. Cat scratch fever can be a serious illness in people, especially those with compromised immune system function, such as individuals undergoing chemotherapy or AIDS patients, the elderly, or children. It causes fever, rashes, and swollen lymph nodes, among other symptoms. *Moraxella bovis* is a bacterium that causes pink eye in both cattle and humans and is common in children who live on ranches or farms.

Exotic pets, including reptiles, birds, and small rodents, can carry dangerous diseases as well, especially when they have been imported from other countries. Rat bite fever and monkey pox are two examples.

In a 2008 survey of 370 veterinarians in Washington state, 280, or about 76 percent, of the respondents recognized that it was very important to educate clients about zoonotic disease prevention. However, only 158, or 43 percent, indicated that they regularly initiated discussions about zoonotic diseases with clients. Only 57 percent had client-education materials on zoonoses available in their clinics. About one-quarter of the veterinarians surveyed had themselves had a zoonotic disease during their careers (Lipton et al. 2008; see also Antech Diagnostics Online 2009).

> *In a 2008 survey of 370 veterinarians in Washington state, 280, or 76 percent, of the respondents recognized that it was very important to educate clients about zoonotic disease prevention. However, only 158, or 43 percent, indicated that they regularly initiated discussions about zoonotic diseases with clients. Only 57 percent had client-education materials on zoonoses available in their clinics.*

External parasites such as fleas, ticks, and sarcoptic mites also affect people. Many times clients find out from their pediatricians that their pets have fleas, because they take their children in to be examined for a rash on the neck, ankles, or arms and discover that it was caused by flea bites. Clients are usually both embarrassed and angry about this state of affairs. Be tactful when dealing with this situation.

Another zoonotic skin problem is ringworm, which can be caused by several species of fungus. Ringworm is usually more of an unsightly, itchy annoyance than a serious disease, but it is very slow to heal and thus not a good thing for clients to get from their new kitten. Skin problems in kittens should always be investigated as soon as possible to prevent the spread of the disease. Ringworm occurs in other species and ages as well, but kittens and barn cats are the most commonly affected pets. Cattle, especially calves, are also common carriers of ringworm.

So how do you communicate to clients about these diseases? The important thing is that you be familiar with them so you know when a warning is needed. When one of these diseases is diagnosed or suspected, clients must be warned that a hazard to their health exists. If you cannot answer all of the client's questions or concerns about the problem, it is imperative to let a doctor or more experienced team member handle the details. The failure of veterinarians to discharge their professional responsibilities with regard to zoonotic diseases can have legal repercussions for the doctor and the practice.

We don't always know when a household with pets also includes an immune-compromised person for whom extra precautions should be taken, and even normal, healthy adults can be affected by zoonotic diseases. It's a good practice to ensure that all clients receive at least some basic information on the topic, such as the handout at the end of this section, so they can protect themselves and their loved ones.

> **COMMON ZOONOTIC DISEASES**
>
> Bartonella (cat scratch fever)
> *E. coli*
> Giardia (camper's diarrhea)
> Hookworms
> Leptospirosis
> Rabies
> Ringworm (dermatophytosis)
> Roundworms
> Salmonella
> Sarcoptes mites (scabies)
> Toxoplasmosis

RESOURCES

American Association of Feline Practitioners. 2003. "Feline Zoonosis Guidelines." www.catvets.com/uploads/PDF/ZooFinal2003.pdf.

"Assessing Client Risk for Zoonotic Disease Transmission." 2008. *Clinician's Brief* 6, no. 4 (April): 21. See the entire issue at www.nxtbook.com/nxtbooks/educationalconcepts/cb_200804/index.php?startid=V8.

Babcock, S., A. E. Marsh, J. Lin, and J. Scott. 2008. "Legal Implications of Zoonoses for Clinical Veterinarians." *Journal of the American Veterinary Medical Association* 233, no. 10 (November): 1576–1586.

Centers for Disease Control and Prevention (CDC), National Center for Infectious Diseases, Division of Parasitic Diseases, in cooperation with the American Association of Veterinary Parasitologists. N.d. "Guidelines for Veterinarians: Prevention of Zoonotic Transmission of Ascarids and Hookworms in Dogs and Cats." www.cdc.gov/ncidod/dpd/parasites/ascaris/prevention.htm. For more information from the CDC for pet owners and veterinary hospitals, see www.cdc.gov/healthypets. Useful CDC publications can also be found at www.cdc.gov/parasites/animal.htm, including "What Every Pet Owner Should Know About Roundworms and Hookworms" (www.cdc.gov/healthypets/Merial_CDCBroch_rsgWEB.pdf); "Toxoplasmosis: An Important Message for Women" (www.cdc.gov/parasites/toxoplasmosis/resources/toxowomen_2.2003.pdf); "Toxoplasmosis: An Important Message for Cat Owners" (www.cdc.gov/parasites/toxoplasmosis/resources/toxo_cat_owners_8-2004.pdf); and "Preventing Infections from Pets: A Guide for People with HIV Infection" (www.cdc.gov/hiv/resources/brochures/pets.htm). For MRSA information from the CDC, see "Community-Associated Methicillin-Resistant *Staphylococcus aureus* (CA-MRSA)" (www.cdc.gov/ncidod/dhqp/ar_mrsa_ca.html) and "Healthcare-Associated Methicillin-Resistant *Staphylococcus aureus* (CA-MRSA)" (www.cdc.gov/ncidod/dhqp/ar_mrsa.html).

Companion Animal Parasite Council, www.capcvet.org. The information on this website covers parasite treatment and prevention protocols. The companion website at www.petsandparasites.org is for pet owners.

Cutler, S. J., A. R. Fooks, and W.H.M. van der Poel. 2010. "Public Health Threat of New, Reemerging and Neglected Zoonoses in the Industrialized World." *Emerging Infectious Diseases* 16, no. 1 (January).

Delta Society, www.deltasociety.org. The Delta Society is a "non-profit organization that helps people live healthier and happier lives by incorporating therapy, service and companion animals into their lives." See the website for more information.

DVM360, www.dvm360.com. DVM360 has several handouts and forms on zoonotic diseases. On the "Business Center" menu, under "Client Handouts," you'll find five handouts under the title "Zoonoses to Know About" and another entitled "Zoonotics: Crucial Questions to Ask Clients During Annual Exams."

Lefebvre, S. L., G. C. Golab, E. Christiansen, et al. 2008. "Guidelines for Animal-Assisted Interventions in Health Care Facilities." *American Journal of Infection Control* 36, no. 2 (March): 78–85.

National Association of State Public Health Veterinarians, www.nasphv.org. The website for this organization gives recommendations on standard infection-control precautions for veterinary personnel and the public. See "The Compendium of Veterinary Standard Precautions for Zoonotic Disease Prevention in Veterinary Personnel," written by the Veterinary Infection Control Committee in 2008, at www.nasphv.org/documents/veterinaryprecautions.pdf, as well as "Model Infection Control Plan for Veterinary Practices," also by the VICC in 2008, at www.nasphv.org/documents/ModelInfectionControlPlan.doc. At www.nasphv.org/documentscompendiumanimals.html, you can download "Animals in Public Settings Compendium" and a users' guide and two posters—"Safety at Animal Exhibits" and "Handwashing."

Rutland, B. R., J. S. Weese, C. Bolin, et al. 2009. "Human-to-Dog Transmission of Methicillin-Resistant *Staphylococcus aureus*" (letter). *Emerging Infectious Diseases* 15, no. 8 (August): 1328–1330.

Weese, J. Scott. 2009. "MRSA: Methicillin-Resistant *Staphylococcus aureus*." VP Client Information Sheets, November 4. www.veterinarypartner.com/Content.plx?P=A&C=15&A=3006&S=0.

ZOONOTIC DISEASES

Pets provide many health benefits to people. Elderly pet owners live longer and make fewer trips to the doctor than those without pets. Children raised with pets become more compassionate adults and are less likely to suffer from pet allergies and asthma. Pets reduce stress and make us laugh at any age.

Despite all these benefits, there is a downside to having pets in the home. Many diseases carried by pets can harm people as well—and vice versa. These diseases are called *zoonoses* (zoo-oh-no-sees). Some of these, such as ringworm, are more annoying than truly harmful, but others, such as rabies, are deadly.

A person's age and health status affect how likely it is that he or she will catch a disease from a pet. The following groups of people may have a compromised immune system and thus be more likely to get sick from an animal-borne disease:

- Infants and children less than five years old
- Elderly people (those over age 70 or so)
- Pregnant women
- People undergoing treatment for cancer (chemotherapy)
- People on immuneosuppressant drugs for organ transplants
- People with HIV/AIDS

If you fit into one of the groups listed above, or a family member or frequent visitor to your home does, you should be extra careful. It is best not to expose an immune-compromised person to high-risk pets. You should also be wary of petting zoos and petting farms.

Some animal species are more likely to transmit diseases than others. These include:

- Reptiles, including turtles, snakes, and lizards
- Baby chicks and ducklings
- Puppies and kittens less than six months old
- Pets with diarrhea or intestinal parasites
- Calves, lambs, and other young farm animals

To prevent illness due to animal contact, the Centers for Disease Control and Prevention (CDC) recommends the following for everyone, but especially for those at greatest risk of getting sick from pets:

- Tell us if someone in your household may be immune-compromised, so that we can advise you on extra precautions that should be taken in particular circumstances.
- In turn, tell us if a human in your household has been diagnosed with any zoonotic disease so that we can monitor or treat your pets as well.

- Always wash your hands thoroughly with soap and running water after contact with animals and their feces.
- Wear gloves to clean soiled litter boxes. If you are pregnant it is best not to clean them at all.
- Keep sandboxes covered to prevent them from being used as litter boxes by stray cats.
- Deworm puppies and kittens according to CDC recommendations.
- Keep puppies and dogs on year-round heartworm preventives, which help prevent roundworm and hookworm transmission to people.
- Have puppies, kittens, and new pets in the household tested for Giardia, a common protozoal parasite that is contagious to dogs, cats, and humans.
- Keep your pets, even indoor ones, vaccinated for rabies.
- Have pets with diarrhea diagnosed and treated promptly.
- Have pets with itching or skin disease diagnosed and treated promptly as well—sarcoptes mites (scabies) and ringworm (a fungal skin infection) are both contagious to people.
- Avoid rough play with cats and dogs to prevent scratches and bites. Have any bite or scratch wound treated promptly. Bartonella (cat scratch fever) is on the rise in the United States and can be deadly to someone with a compromised immune system.
- Never leave children alone or unsupervised with a pet. Most dog-bite injuries occur in children less than five years of age.

CONCLUDING THOUGHTS

Medicine has become so complex over the years, and there are so many things to teach ourselves and our clients, that I wish the alphabet were a whole lot longer. There are so many topics that I could not cover, or that I barely touched upon—alternative medicine, dermatology, feline care, and rehabilitation, to name a few. Luckily, the communication principles outlined at the beginning of this book can be applied to almost any aspect of veterinary care.

The role of the veterinarian and the veterinary team has changed, too. In the historical view, veterinarians protected human health by improving the health of farm animals and preventing the spread of disease from animals to humans. This is still true today, but veterinarians also now protect people against another plague—loneliness. In recent years, human medicine has recognized that lack of social support, depression, and loneliness are strongly associated with serious medical problems, including heart disease and cancer. The influence of loneliness may be as great a risk factor as smoking and cholesterol levels.

Companion animals are considered family members by most of their owners and are one of society's major bulwarks against loneliness and depression. Nurturing animals contributes to people's emotional equilibrium. We are privileged in this profession to contribute not just to the health of animals but to the health of pet owners.

My chapter on zoonotic diseases notwithstanding, it is much more important to communicate to your clients how good pets are for people than it is to warn them of the dangers of pet ownership. Pets help people live longer, happier lives. Ninety-four percent of people hospitalized after a heart attack who happened to own pets were still alive one year later, compared with only 72 percent of those who did not own pets. Of nearly 1,000 institutionalized older adult Medicare patients, those who owned pets appeared to experience less distress and required fewer visits to their physicians than those who did not own pets. Married couples with pets have fewer arguments and get divorced less often. Pets have been shown to help lower blood pressure, help older adults and people with special needs function better and live longer, provide a healthy link with nature, boost morale, and provide companionship that may be lacking in busy or lonely lives. Interacting with a pet involves our sense of touch in a way that reduces stress—what could be better than snuggling with an affectionate dog or cat? Pets are the best prescription for a long and happy life.

Pets remind us of what it is to be wild, gentle, and loyal—to trust, to flourish, and to slow down with age. Eventually, they teach us how to let go and say good-bye. They make us laugh and they help us through hard times. They teach our children compassion and they keep us company when we grow old. For all that our pets give us, for all the love and joy they bring to our lives, we can be grateful, and grateful too for the chance we have to be their caretakers.

There is no better job on earth than one that lets us celebrate and cherish the bond between people and their pets, giving us so much opportunity to improve the lives of both our clients and our patients. Make the most of this precious gift and teach your clients well; their lives, as well as those of their pets, may depend on it!

REFERENCES

Alef, M., F. von Praun, and G. Oechtering. 2008. "Is Routine Pre-Anesthetic Haematologic and Biochemical Screening Justified in Dogs?" *Veterinary Anaesthesia and Analgesia* 35: 132–140.

American Academy of Periodontology (AAP). N.d. "Mouth-Body Connection." http://www.perio.org/consumer/mbc.top2.htm.

Antech Diagnostics Online. 2009. "Legal and Prevention Issues of Zoonoses." March. http://www.antechdiagnostics.com/antech1.shtml?n=r&p=newsletter0309a.

Armstrong, P. J., E. M. Lund, C. A. Kirk, et al. 2004. "Prevalence and Risk Factors for Obesity in Dogs and Cats." *Proceedings of the American College of Veterinary Internal Medicine* 22: 6–7.

Aucoin, D. 2006. *An Analysis of Canine and Feline Wellness Profiles in Young Adults: The Case for Early Detection of Chronic Disease*. Antech Laboratories.

Beaver, B. V. 1999. *Canine Behavior: A Guide for Veterinarians*. Philadelphia: W. B Saunders.

Beaver, B. V., and L. I. Haug. 2003. "Canine Behaviors Associated with Hypothyroidism." *Journal of the American Animal Hospital Association* 39: 431–434.

Bertone, E. R., L. A. Snyder, and A. S. Moore. 2003. "Environmental and Lifestyle Risk Factors for Oral Squamous Cell Carcinoma in Domestic Cats." *Journal of Veterinary Internal Medicine* 17: 557–562.

———. 2002. "Environmental Tobacco Smoke and Risk of Malignant Lymphoma in Pet Cats." *American Journal of Epidemiology* 156: 268–273.

Blagburn, B. L., D. S. Lindsay, J. L. Vaughan, et al. 1996. "Prevalence of Canine Parasites Based on Fecal Flotation." *Compendium of Continuing Education for Practicing Veterinarians* 18, no. 5: 483–509.

Burkholder, W. J. 2001. "Precision and Practicality of Methods Assessing Body Composition of Dogs and Cats." *Compendium of Continuing Education for Practicing Veterinarians* 23: 1–10.

Catanzaro, T. 1996. *Building the Successful Veterinary Practice*, vol. 2: *Programs and Procedures*. Golden, CO: Catanzaro and Associates.

Centers for Disease Control and Prevention (CDC). 2009. "Dog Bite Prevention." www.cdc.gov/ncipc/duip/biteprevention.htm.

Chastain, C. B., and D. Panciera. 2003. "Neutering-Induced Changes in Plasma Insulin Concentrations in Cats." *Small Animal Clinical Endocrinology* 13, no. 2: 40–41.

Chastain, C. B., D. Panciera, and C. Waters. 1999. "Associations Between Age, Parity, Hormonal Therapy and Breed, and Pyometra in Finnish Dogs." *Small Animal Endocrinology* 9: 8.

"Chemical Levels High in Pets." 2008. *Veterinary Forum*. May 24.

Clarke, S. P., and D. Bennett. 2006. "Feline Osteoarthritis: A Prospective Study of 28 Cases." *Journal of Small Animal Practice* 47: 439–445.

Committee on Health Literacy, Board on Neuroscience and Behavioral Health, and Institute of Medicine of the National Academies. 2004. *Health Literacy: A Prescription to End*

Confusion. Lynn Nielsen-Bohlman, Allison M. Panzer, and David A. Kindig, eds. Washington, DC: National Academies Press.

ConsumerLab.com. 2009a. "Contamination and Mislabeling Discovered in over 20% of Arthritis Supplements Selected for Review." Initial posting July 6, 2009, updated August 2, 2010. https://www.consumerlab.com/reviews/Joint_Supplements_Glucosamine_Chondroitin_MSM_Review/jointsupplements/.

———. 2009b. "Joint Pain Supplements for Dogs, Cats, and Horses Often Lack Key Ingredient." Initial posting July 6, 2009, updated August 2, 2010. https://www.consumerlab.com/reviews/Joint_Supplements_Glucosamine_Chondroitin_and_MSM_Dogs_Cats_Horses/jointsupplements_pets/.

Cooley, D. M., B. C. Beranek, D. L. Schkittler, et al. 2002. "Endogenous Gonadal Hormone Exposure and Bone Sarcoma Risk." *Cancer Epidemiology, Biomarkers and Prevention* 11, no. 11: 1434–1440.

Cupp, C. J., W. W. Kerr, J. P. Clementine, et al. 2008. "The Role of Nutritional Interventions in the Longevity and Maintenance of Long-Term Health in Aging Cats." *International Journal of Applied Research in Veterinary Medicine* 6: 34–50.

Cutler, S. J., A. R. Fooks, and W.H.M. van der Poel. 2010. "Public Health Threat of New, Reemerging and Neglected Zoonoses in the Industrialized World." *Emerging Infectious Diseases* 12: 1–7.

Dale, Edgar. 1969. *Audio-Visual Methods in Technology,* 3rd ed. Austin, TX: Holt, Rinehart and Winston.

Debowes, L. 1992. "Systemic Effects of Oral Disease." *AVDC/AVD* [American Veterinary Dental College/Academy of Veterinary Dentistry] *Proceedings* 65.

DeBowes, L. J., D. Mosier, E. Logan, et al. 1996. In "The Association of Periodontal Disease and Histologic Lesions in Multiple Organs from 45 Dogs." *Journal of Veterinary Dentistry* 13: 57–60.

Donaghue, S., and D. Dzanis. 1995. "Evaluating Commercial Diets." In *Association of Reptilian and Amphibian Veterinarians Proceedings,* Second Annual Conference, October 27–29, Sacramento, CA, pp. 74–79.

Downs, J. S., W. Bruine de Bruine, and B. Fischoff. 2008. "Parents' Vaccination Comprehension and Decisions." *Vaccine* 26: 1595–1607.

Dye, J. A., M. Venier, L. Zhu, et al. 2007. "Elevated PBDE Levels in Cats: Sentinels for Humans?" *Environmental Science and Technology* 41, no. 18: 6350–6356.

Dzanis, D. A. 1994a. "The Association of American Feed Control Officials Dog and Cat Food Nutrient Profiles: Substantiation of Nutritional Adequacy of Complete and Balanced Pet Foods in the United States." *Journal of Nutrition* 124: 2535S–2539S.

———. 1994b. "Regulation of Health Claims for Pet Foods." *Veterinary Clinical Nutrition* 1: 5–11.

Edney, A. T., and P. M. Smith. 1986. "Study of Obesity in Dogs Visiting Veterinary Practices in the United Kingdom." *Veterinary Record* 118, no. 14: 391–396.

Elliott, J., J. M. Rawlings, P. J. Markwell, and P. J. Barber. 2000. "Survival of Cats with Naturally Occurring Renal Failure: Effect of Dietary Management." *Journal of Small Animal Practice* 41, no. 6: 235–242.

Eskeland, G. E., R. H. Tilung, and M. Baken. 2007. "The Importance of Consistency in the Training of Dogs: The Effect of Punishment, Rewards, Control and Attitude on Obedience and Problem Behaviours in Dogs." In G. Landsberg, S. Matiello, and D. Mills, eds., *Proceedings of the Sixth International Veterinary Behaviour and European College of Veterinary Behavioural Medicine—Companion Animals.* Birmingham, UK: European Society of Veterinary Clinical Ethology.

Francis, D. P., S. M. Cotter, W. D. Hardy Jr., et al. 1979. "Comparison of Virus-Positive and Virus-Negative Cases of Feline Leukemia and Lymphoma." *Cancer Research* 39: 3866–3870.

Freeman, L. M., S. K. Abood, A. J. Fascetti, et al. 2006. "Disease Prevalence Among Dogs and Cats in the United States and Australia and Proportions of Dogs and Cats That Receive Therapeutic Diets or Dietary Supplements." *Journal of the American Veterinary Medical Association* 229, no. 4: 531–534.

Freeman, L. M., and D. E. Linder. 2010. "An Evaluation of Calorie Density and Feeding Directions for Commercially Available Weight-Control Diets." *Journal of the American Veterinary Medical Association* 236, no. 1: 74–77.

Fujimura, T., T. Matsumoto, S. Tanabe, et al. 2008. "Specific Discrimination of Chicken DNA from Other Poultry DNA in Processed Foods Using the Polymerase Chain Reaction." *Bioscience, Biotechnology, and Biochemistry* 72, no. 3: 909–913.

George, L. K. 2006. "Perceived Quality of Life." In R. H. Binstock and L. K. George, eds., *Handbook of Aging and the Social Sciences*, 6th ed. San Diego: Elsevier.

German, A. J. 2006. "The Growing Problem of Obesity in Dogs and Cats." *Journal of Nutrition* 136: 1940S–1946S.

Glickman, L. T., M. Raghaven, D. W. Knapp, et al. 2004. "Herbicide Exposure and the Risk of Transitional Cell Carcinoma of the Urinary Bladder in Scottish Terriers." *Journal of the American Veterinary Medical Association* 224, no. 8: 1290–1297.

Gorbach, S. L. 2000. "Probiotics and Gastrointestinal Health." *American Journal of Gastroenterology* 95 (Supplement): S1–S4.

Hand, M. S., D. Craig, R. L. Thatcher, et al. 2010. *Small Animal Clinical Nutrition*, 5th ed. Topeka, KS: Mark Morris Institute.

Hardie, E., S. Roe, and F. Martin. 2002. "Radiographic Evidence of Degenerative Joint Disease in Geriatric Cats: 100 Cases (1994–1997)." *Journal of the American Veterinary Medical Association* 220: 628–632.

Hawk, T. F., and A. J. Shah. 2007. "Using Learning Style Instruments to Enhance Student Learning." *Decision Sciences Journal of Innovative Education* 5, no. 1: 1–19.

Herrmann, N., L. T. Glickman, P. M. Schantz, et al. 1985. "Seroprevalence of Zoonotic Toxocariasis in the United States: 1971–1973." *American Journal of Epidemiology* 122, no. 5: 890–896.

Herron, M., F. Shofer, and I. Reisner. 2009. "Survey of the Use and Outcome of Confrontational and Non-Confrontational Training Methods in Client-Owned Dogs Showing Undesired Behaviors." *Applied Animal Behavior Science* 117, nos. 1–2: 47–54.

Hielm-Bjorkman, A. K., E. Kuusela, A. Liman, et al. 2003. "Evaluation of Methods for Assessment of Pain Associated with Chronic Osteoarthritis in Dogs." *Journal of the American Veterinary Medical Association* 222: 1552–1558.

Impellizeri, J. A., M. A. Tetrick, and P. Muir. 2000. "Effect of Weight Reduction on Clinical Signs of Lameness in Dogs with Hip Dysplasia." *Journal of the American Veterinary Medical Association* 216: 1089–1091.

Jevring, Caroline, and Tom Catanzaro. 1999. *Healthcare of the Well Pet*. Philadelphia: W. B. Saunders.

Jonker, K. M., J.J.H.C. Tilburg, G. H. Hagele, et al. 2008. "Species Identification in Meat Products Using Real-Time PCR." *Food Additives and Contaminants: Part A—Chemistry, Analysis, Control, Exposure and Risk Assessment* 25, no. 5: 527–533.

Kahn A., P. Bauche, and J. Lamoureux. 2003. "Child Victims of Dog Bites Treated in Emergency Departments: A Prospective Survey." *European Journal of Pediatrics* 162, no. 4: 254–258.

Kazacos, K. 2004. "Pets, Parasites and People: A Roundtable on Zoonotic Disease." *Veterinary Forum* 20(A): 1–16.

Kealy, R. D., D. F. Lawler, J. M. Ballam, et al. 2002. "Influence of Diet Restriction on Life Span and Age-Related Changes in Labrador Retrievers." *Journal of the American Veterinary Medical Association* 220: 1315–1320.

Kitchell, B. 2007. "Feline Oncology: What's New." AAHA Annual Meeting, March, Denver, CO.

Kolars, J., L. Gruppen, P. Traber, et al. 1997. "The Effect of Student- and Teacher-Centred Small-Group Learning in Medical School on Knowledge Acquisition, Retention, and Application." *Medical Teacher* 19, no. 1: 53–57.

Kolb, D. 1984. *Experiential Learning: Experience as the Source of Learning and Development.* Englewood Cliffs, NJ: Prentice Hall.

Laflamme, D. P. 2007. "Obesity: What Is It Really? *Nestle Purina Research Report* 11, no. 2: 2–4.

Lana, S. E., L. R. Kogan, J. R. Graham, and N. G. Robinson. 2006. "The Use of Complementary and Alternative Therapies in Dogs and Cats with Cancer." *Journal of the American Animal Hospital Association* 42: 361–365.

Lawler, D. F., R. H. Evans, B. T. Larson, et al. 2005. "Influence of Lifetime Food Restriction on Causes, Time, and Predictors of Death in Dogs." *Journal of the American Veterinary Medical Association* 226: 225–231.

"Learning Retention Rate." N.d. www.tenouk.com/learningretentionrate.html.

Lewis, H. B. 2006. "Healthy Pets Benefit from Blood Work." *Banfield* 2: 18–20.

Lipton, B. A., S. G. Hopkins, J. E. Koehler, et al. 2008. "A Survey of Veterinarian Involvement in Zoonotic Disease Prevention Practices." *Journal of the American Veterinary Medical Association* 233: 1242–1249.

Little, S. 2004. "Parasites and People: A Roundtable on Zoonotic Disease." *Veterinary Forum* 20(A): 1–16.

Loesche, E. J. 1994. "Periodontal Disease as a Risk Factor for Heart Disease." *Compendium* 15: 976, 978–982.

Lund, E. M., P. J. Armstrong, C. A. Kirk, and J. S. Klausner. 2006. "Prevalence and Risk Factors for Obesity in Adult Dogs from Private U.S. Veterinary Practices." *International Journal of Applied Research in Veterinary Medicine* 3, no. 2: 88–96.

Lund, E. M., P. J. Armstrong, C. A. Kirk, L. M. Kolar, and J. S. Klausner. 1999. "Health Status and Population Characteristics of Dogs and Cats Examined at Private Veterinary Practices in the United States." *Journal of the American Veterinary Medical Association* 214, no. 9: 1336–1341.

Mawby, D. I., J. W. Bartges, A. d'Avignon, et al. 2004. "Comparison of Various Methods for Estimating Body Fat in Dogs." *Journal of the American Animal Hospital Association* 40: 109–114.

McGreevy, P. D., P. C. Thomson, C. Pride, et al. 2005. "Prevalence of Obesity in Dogs Examined by Australian Veterinary Practices and the Risk Factors Involved." *Veterinary Record* 156, no. 22: 695–702.

Monroy, A., P. Behar, M. Nagy, et al. 2009. "Head and Neck Bites in Children." *Otolaryngology—Head and Neck Surgery* 140: 354–357.

National Council on Pet Population Study and Policy. N.d. "Shelter Statistics Survey, 1994–1997." http://www.petpopulation.org/statsurvey.html.

New, J. C., W. J. Kelch, J. M. Hutchison, et al. 2004. "Birth and Death Rate Estimates of Cats and Dogs in U.S. Households and Related Factors." *Journal of Applied Animal Welfare Science* 7, no. 4: 229–241.

Nguyen, P. G., H. J. Dumon, B. S. Siliart, et al. 2004. "Effects of Dietary Fat and Energy on Body Weight and Composition After Gonadectomy in Cats." *American Journal of Veterinary Research* 65, no. 12: 1708–1713.

Oglesbee, Barbara L. 2006. *The 5-Minute Veterinary Consult: Ferret and Rabbit*. New York: Blackwell.

Patronek, G. J., L. T. Glickman, A. M. Beck, et al. 1996. "Risk Factors for the Relinquishment of Dogs to an Animal Shelter." *Journal of the American Veterinary Medical Association* 209, no. 3: 572–581.

Peterson, M. C., J. Holbrook, D. Von Hales, et al. 1992. "Contributions of the History, Physical Examination and Laboratory Investigation in Making Medical Diagnoses." *Western Journal of Medicine* 156: 163–165.

Peterson, N. 2007. "Degenerative Joint Disease in Cats." *Veterinary Practice News*. August.

Plantinga, E. A., H. Everts, A. M. Kastelein, and A. C. Beynen. 2005. "Retrospective Study of the Survival of Cats with Acquired Chronic Renal Insufficiency Offered Different Commercial Diets." *Veterinary Record* 157, no. 7: 185–187.

Raghaven, M., D. W. Knapp, M. H. Dawson, et al. 2004. "Topical Flea and Tick Pesticides and the Risk of Transitional Cell Carcinoma of the Urinary Bladder in Scottish Terriers." *Journal of the American Veterinary Medical Association* 225, no. 3: 389–394.

Reisner, I. R., F. S. Shofer, and M. L. Nance. 2007. "Behavioral Assessment of Child-Directed Canine Aggression." *Injury Prevention* 13, no. 5: 348–351.

Rusk, A. W., and C. Khanna. 2005. "Cancer: Cases Likely Will Rise in Aging Animals." *DVM Newsmagazine*. March.

Rutlan, B. R., J. S. Weese, C. Bolin, et al. 2009. "Human-to-Dog Transmission of Methicillin-Resistant *Staphylococcus aureus*" (letter). *Emerging Infectious Diseases* 15: 1328–1330.

Scarlett, J. M., and S. Donaghue. 1998. "Associations Between Body Condition and Disease in Cats." *Journal of the American Veterinary Medical Association* 212: 1725–1731.

———. 1994. "Overweight Cats: Prevalence and Risk Factors." *International Journal of Obesity* 18: S22–S28.

Scarlett, J. M., M. D. Salman, J. G. New, and P. H. Kass. 2002. "The Role of Veterinary Practitioners in Reducing Dog and Cat Relinquishments and Euthanasias." *Journal of the American Veterinary Medical Association* 220, no. 3: 306–311.

Schantz, P. M., A. R. Moorhead, et al. 1994. "Intestinal Parasites Are Common in Fulton County, Georgia." In *Proceedings of the Annual Meeting of the American Association of Veterinary Parasitology*, no. 80. San Francisco: AAVP.

Schwartz, M. A. 1995. *Listen to Me, Doctor: Taking Charge of Your Own Health Care*. San Francisco: MacAdam/Cage.

Semb, J., and J. Ellis. 1994. "Knowledge Taught in School: What Is Remembered?" *Review of Educational Research* 64, no. 2: 253–286.

Shuler, C. M., E. E. DeBess, J. A. Lapidus, and K. Hedberg. 2008. "Canine and Human Factors Related to Dog Bite Injuries." *Journal of the American Veterinary Medical Association* 232, no. 4: 542–546.

Silverberg, J., A. Taylor-Vaisey, J. Szalai, and J. Tipping. 1995. "Lectures, Interactive Learning, and Knowledge Retention in Continuing Medical Education." *Journal of Continuing Education in the Health Professions* 15, no. 4: 231–234.

Sisson, J., R. Swartz, and F. Wolf. 1992. "Learning, Retention and Recall of Clinical Information." *Medical Education* 26, no. 6: 454–461.

Sutton, N. M., N. Bates, and A. Campbell. 2007. "Clinical Effects and Outcomes of Feline Permethrin Spot-on Poisonings Reported to the Veterinary Poisons Information Service (VPIS), London." *Journal of Feline Medicine and Surgery* 9: 335–339.

Tilley, L. P., and F.W.K. Smith Jr. 2008. *Blackwell's Five-Minute Veterinary Consult: Canine and Feline*, 4th ed. New York: Blackwell.

Torpy, J. M., A. E. Burke, and R. M. Glass. 2008. "Periodontal Disease." *Journal of the American Medical Association* 299, no. 5: 598.

Trayhurn, P. 2006. "Inflammation in Obesity: Down to the Fat?" *Compendium on Continuing Education for the Practicing Veterinarian* 28 (Supplement 4A): 33–36.

Trayhurn, P., and I. S. Wood. 2005. "Signaling Role of Adipose Tissue: Adipokines and Inflammation in Obesity." *Biochemical Society Transaction* 33, no. 5: 1078–1081.

Tremayne, Jessica. 2010. "Therapeutic Diets." *Veterinary Practice News*. http://www.veterinarypracticenews.com/vet-dept/small-animal-dept/therapeutic-diets.aspx.

Van Wessum, R., C. E. Harvey, and P. Hennet. 1992. "Feline Dental Resorptive Lesions: Prevalence Patterns." *Veterinary Clinics of North America: Small Animal Practice* 22: 1405–1416.

Weese, J. S., and L. Arroyo. 2003. "Bacteriological Evaluation of Dog and Cat Diets That Claim to Contain Probiotics." *Canadian Veterinary Journal* 44: 212–215.

Wiggs, R. B., and H. B. Loprise. 1997. "Veterinary Dentistry Principles and Practice." Philadelphia: Lippincott-Raven.

Wise, J. K., and J. J. Yang. 1994. "Dog and Cat Ownership, 1991–1998." *Journal of the American Veterinary Medical Association* 204: 1166–1167.

Wiseman-Orr, M. L., E. M. Scott, J. Reid, et al. 2006. "Validation of a Structured Questionnaire as an Instrument to Measure Chronic Pain in Dogs on the Basis of Effects on Health-Related Quality of Life." *American Journal of Veterinary Research* 67: 1826–1836.

INDEX

Advocate, serving as, xxx–xxxi, 7, 19, 25, 71, 92
Aggression, 6, 9, 161
Allergic bronchitis, 63
Allergies, 37, 116
American Animal Hospital Association (AAHA), 6, 100, 177, 189; Compliance Study by, vi; Helping Pets Fund of, 108
American Association of Feline Practitioners (AAFP), 63, 81
American Heartworm Society (AHS), 59, 60, 61, 63
American Veterinary Dental College (VOHC), 29
American Veterinary Medical Association, 134
Anaplasmosis, 49
Anemia, 43, 90, 93
Anesthesia, xx, xxi, 20, 26, 30, 31, 35, 124, 143, 163, 164, 168, 177, 207, 213, 214; consent forms for, 32; deaths under, 103, 157; dental cleaning and, 172; estimates for, 105, 110–111; fear of, 179; monitoring, 176; problems from, 157, 179; procedures for, 104, 162; safe, 104, 159, 166
Anterior cruciate ligament (ACL), 73
Antibiotics, 103, 104, 159, 172, 205
Antioxidants, 118, 217
Appointments, viii, xv, 1–4, 100–101, 107; scheduling, 2–3, 4, 143, 175, 177
Arthritis, 9, 71, 72, 120, 132, 151, 181, 197, 201, 217; graphic depiction of, 75; joint injury and, 73; obesity and, 217; progression of, 74, 75; risk of, 198; score card, 76; spinal, 73
Association for Pet Obesity Prevention (APOP), 197
Asthma, 63
Authorization for treatment forms, 34–35, 39
Average transaction fee (ATF), vii

Bacterial infections, 223, 224
Bad news, delivering, 30, 32
Bartonella, 224, 225
Bathing, 84, 216–217
Behavior, xxvi, 5–10, 80, 192, 211; assertive, 39; changes in, 217; finicky, 116; inherited, 78; knowledge base in, 9; urinary, 181, 182, 183
Behavior problems, 5, 7, 8, 9, 81, 149; solving, 184–185
Billing, xiii, xix, 31, 107
Bites, 5, 8, 81, 193
Biting insects, 43–51
Bladder infections, 9, 181
Bladder stones, 90, 152, 171, 182
Blood-clotting disorders, 163
Blood oxygen level, 207
Blood pressure, 132, 207, 213, 232; monitoring, 150, 214
Blood samples, 150, 172, 206
Blood testing, 19, 64, 80, 89, 91, 102, 117, 160, 181, 223; pre-anesthetic, xii, xxv, 27, 32, 83, 85, 90, 92, 106, 176, 177, 206

Boarding, 203, 204
Body language/posture, xix, xv, xxxvii, 106
Bordetella, 82, 104, 151, 191
Brochures, xxviii, 134, 172, 175, 203
Brucellosis, 160
Buccal bleeding time (BBT), 163

Cancer, vii, 15–21, 29, 149, 150, 198, 201, 231; diagnosis of, 15–16, 21; diet and, 116; mammary, 160; markers for, 90; preventing, 15, 16, 23–24; prostatic, 161; screening tests for, 23; side effects of, 20; testicular, 161; treating, 16, 17, 18, 19, 21
Cardiomyopathy, 90, 151
Cardiovascular disease, 217
Care, xxi, xxiv, xxxii, xxxiii, xxxiv, 5, 78, 123, 141, 142, 185, 196, 204, 205, 231; behavioral, 190; compromising, 103; costs of, 39, 209–210; ear, 104, 211; emergency, 39–40, 100; estimates for, 101, 103; follow-up, 104; home, 27–28, 29, 163; hospice, 17; hospital, 2; knowledge of, xxiii, xxxi, 127; nutritional, 190; offering, xxxi; outpatient, 102; post-surgical, 169; preventive, 190, 195, 212; pro bono, 100, 108; quality, ix, 208, 212; refusing, xx, 27–28, 179; senior pet, 211–218; teaching, vi, xxix; wellness, xxxi, 93, 151, 212, 213, 214
CareCredit, 100, 178
Cat fleas (*Ctenocephalides felis*), 43
Cat scratch fever, 224, 225
Catanzaro, Tom, 142
Cats International, handouts by, 183
Centers for Disease Control and Prevention (CDC), 5, 49, 82, 84, 193, 228
Chemistry, 92, 150
Chemotherapy, 17, 20, 21, 224
Chew toys, 29, 32, 83
Chewing, 5, 8, 80, 217
Cheyletiella mites, 50

Chlorhexidine mouth rinse, 28, 29
Chondroitin sulfate, 119
Client relations specialists (CRS), vi, xxxii, xxxiii, 53, 54, 142
Clients: arguing with, 108, 172; bonding with, xxvii, 38, 85; education of, xii, xiii, xxvi, xxix, xxxii, 80, 149–150, 151, 153, 192, 204, 212, 214; grieving, 53–56; listening to, xix–xx, 72; new, 100–101; payments and, 104–105; questioning, 139–143; recruiting, xix, 2, 208; retaining, xix, xxv; supervising, xx–xxi; types of, xiv–xv, xxv
Coagulopathy, 104
Colitis, diet and, 116
Communication, v, xviii, xiv, xix–xx, 9, 50, 143, 144; auditory, xxii; education and, xxxii; effective, vi–vii, viii, xxix; emergencies and, 41; importance of, 132, 216; improving, xiii, xxviii; kinesthetic, xxii–xxiii; listening and, xxxiii; maxims for, xi–xxxii; money matters and, 99; nonverbal, xxxiv; post–surgical, 162, 163; principles of, xxxvii, 231; team, xii–xiv; telephone, 171–179; visual, xxii
Companion Animal Parasite Council (CAPC), 82, 84
Complete blood count (CBC), 49, 50, 90, 91, 104, 132; baseline, 94; results for, 96
Compliance, xxxii, xxxvi, 67, 215
Compliance Study (AAHA), vi
Counseling, 8, 79, 204, 212
Cremation, 53, 55
Cryptosporidium, 223
Cushing's disease, xxvi
Customer service, xix, 1

Dale, Edgar, xxiv
Death, coping with, xxi, xxvi, 54, 55, 56
Decision making, xxxiv, 17–21, 42, 167; pet-care, 85, 90, 102, 103, 129

Declawing, 84, 85, 183
Defecation, problems with, 182, 184
Degenerative joint disease (DJD), 71, 72, 73
Dehydration, 17, 90
Demodectic mites, 50
Dental care, vi, xxi, xxiii, xxiv–xxv, xxxii, 32, 83, 84, 103, 142, 150, 151, 160, 192, 211, 212; anesthesia and, 172; cost of, 27, 31; health plan for, 30; home, 28, 29; importance of, 25; life expectancy and, 29; reminders about, 178; scheduling, 27, 179
Dental disease, 149, 151, 172, 217; seriousness of, xxi–xxii
Dentistry, 25–32, 34, 151, 204, 205
Depression, xviii, 231
Dermatology, 231
Dermatophytosis, 225
Deworming, 66, 67, 84
Diabetes, vii, xxxv, 17, 90, 93, 141, 181, 198, 201, 213
Diagnoses, xx, xxvi, xxxii, xxxiii, xxxvi, 89, 139, 140, 213
Diarrhea, xxxii, 16, 17, 45, 62, 66, 67, 116, 120, 225
Diet, 141, 153, 218; cancer and, 23; changing, 32, 114, 115–116, 117; high-quality, 23; low-calorie, 199; prescription, 120; tarter-control, 29; therapeutic, vi, 116, 117–118, 200
Diseases, 38, 100, 153, 192, 224; categorizing, 150; contagious, 80; explaining, xxxv, xxxvii; frequency of, 150; infectious, 149; insect-borne, 49; risk of, 79, 212; senior pets and, 213; treating, 140, 232
Distemper: cat/dog, 189, 190; vaccination for, 173, 175, 189, 194, 198
Distemper-hepatitis-leptospirosis-parainfluenza-parvovirus (DHLPP), 82
Distemper-hepatitis-parainfluenza-parvovirus (DHPP), 82
Dry eye (KCS), 150, 214
Dry skin, diet and, 116

Dysplasia, 73, 152, 163
E. coli, 223, 225
Ear infections, 29, 151, 205
Ear-mites, 207
Ebola virus, 221
Education, vii, xiv, xxi, 80, 123, 200; client, vi, xi, xii, xxvi, xxix, xxxii, 149–150, 151, 192, 204, 212, 214; continuing, viii, xviii; public, 46; types of, xxxii–xxxvii
Ehrlichiosis, 49
Electrocardiograms (ECGs), 32, 89, 90, 94, 103, 104, 142, 151, 152, 157, 160, 172, 179, 203, 206, 208, 213, 214
Emergencies, 37–42, 100, 204, 213; communication and, 41; empathy in, 37; handling, 38–40; payments and, 107
Empathy, xxxiii, xxxiv, xxxvi, 30, 56, 125, 173; cancer and, 20; emergencies and, 37
Endoscopy, 207
Engage, xxx–xxxiv
Enlist, xxxiii, xxxvi–xxxvii
Enthusiasm, expressing, xxi–xxii, 77, 176
Environmental Protection Agency (EPA), 45, 46
Enzyme-linked immunosorbant assay (ELISA), 90
Equipment, 89, 90, 203, 205–206, 207, 208
Estimates, 99, 100, 101–106; form for, 110–111
Euthanasia, 20, 39, 41, 51, 53–56, 74, 81, 100, 159, 161, 184; appointments for, 3; behavior problems and, 5; payment for, 56
Exams, vii, xxxiv, 28, 32, 80, 151, 191, 192, 195; yearly, 211–218
Exercise, 153, 197–202, 213
Eye diseases, 150

Fatty acids, 118, 120, 123, 217
Fear, as adaptive trait, 8
Fecal centrifugation, 82, 83, 84
Feces, 67, 123; picking up/disposing of, 68

Feline Handling Guidelines (AAFP), 81
Feline Idiopathic Cystitis (FIC), 181
Feline immunodeficiency virus (FIV), 24, 80, 84, 161, 191, 192, 212
Feline infectious peritonitis (FIP), xxvi, 80, 212
Feline leukemia virus (FeLV), xii, 24, 80, 84, 89, 105, 161, 191, 192
Feline lower urinary tract disease (FLUTD), 84, 116
Feline viral rhinotracheitis-calicivirus-chlamydia-panleukopenia (FVRCCP), 84
Flea products, 45–46, 47, 50, 124, 140
Fleas, 43–51, 221, 224; bites from, 50, 225; controlling, xxv, 43, 45, 46–47, 48, 49, 50, 56, 68, 211; fascinating facts about, 44
Food charts, sample entries for, 118
Formalin, 65
Fungus, 50, 225

Gastrointestinal disease, 66, 139, 222
Gastrointestinal (GI) system, 114, 146–147
Genetic disorders, 90, 152, 163, 182
Genetics, 21, 120, 149, 152, 212
Giardia, 66, 68, 83, 222, 225
Gingivitis, 26, 32, 217
Glaucoma, 214
Glucosamine, 118, 119, 140
Goals, xii, xiii, xxxvii, 126, 204, 215, 216
Goethe, Johann Wolfgang von: quote of, xiv
Golden Rule, xiv–xv, 38, 56
Grief counseling, 39, 53–56
Grooming, 8, 44, 84, 192, 216, 217

Handouts, xv, xxiii, xxvi–xxix, xxx, 6, 7, 17, 39, 83, 85, 92, 129, 183, 204, 205; appropriate, 79 cancer-prevention, 150; presurgery, 160
Health care, vi, xxxiv, 2, 8, 77, 92, 212; dealing with, xxxvi; literacy, xxxv; plans, 99, 101, 191–192, 211; promoting, 176
Heart attacks, 30, 231
Heart disease, 17, 63, 89, 90, 116, 132, 152, 198, 201, 205, 231
Heartworm associated respiratory disease (HARD), 63
Heartworm disease, xxv, xxxvii, 49, 61, 67, 190; medication for, xxxvi, 62, 63–64, 82, 83, 84, 85, 101, 131, 140, 175; testing for, 2, 3, 49, 60, 61, 80, 101, 104
Heartworms, xxii, 59–64, 68
Helping Pets Fund (AAHA), 108
Hematocrit, 90, 96
Hepatic lipidosis, vii, 198
Hepatic microdysplasia, 163
Hepatitis, 91, 152, 217
Histopathology, 104
History taking, 140–141, 145, 146–147
Honesty, importance of, xx–xxi, 20, 31, 40–41, 55, 102, 108, 124
Hookworms, 65, 66, 68, 222, 223, 225
Housetraining, 83, 175, 182, 184, 192
Humane Society, 82, 84, 130, 181, 184
Hypertension, 213
Hyperthyroidism, xxvi, 81, 213
Hypertrophy, 161

Immunity, 190, 224, 225
Incontinence, 132, 181
Inflammatory bowel disease, 120
Influenza, 191, 221
Information, xxvi, xxvii, xxx, 20, 41, 72, 129, 160, 175, 194, 204–205, 215; background, 182; collecting, 139, 140, 142, 153, 213; confusing/conflicting, 21; dealing with, xxxiii, xxxvi; emergencies and, 37; medication, 130; objective, 139, 140; processing, xxxv; sharing, 18, 31, 139, 171; sources of, 6, 78; subjective, 139, 140
Insecticides, 47, 48, 50
Institute for Safe Medication Practices (ISMP), 130

Institute of Medicine, xxxv
Insulin, xxxv, xxxvii
Insurance, 99, 100, 181
Internet, vi, xxvi, 101, 132, 194
Intraocular pressure (IOP), 214
Invoices, presenting, 100, 106–108
Isofluorane, 124

Joint disease, 71–75, 198

Kidney disease, 17, 72, 81, 89, 90, 92, 93, 141, 150, 172, 181, 201, 213, 217, 218, 224; diet and, 115, 116, 118; monitoring, 132
Kidney stones, 181
Kittens, caring for, 77–85

Laboratory tests, xxxiv, 89–93
Lameness, 16, 72, 73, 222
Learning, different ways of, xxii–xxiii, 26, 134
Leptospirosis, 224, 225
Lice, 50
Life expectancy, vii, 17, 27, 182, 197, 202, 212, 218; dental care and, 29; happiness and, xvii–xviii
Listening, xix–xx, 72, 139, 140, 142; communication and, xxxiii
Litter-box problems, 8, 73, 81, 183, 186, 187, 223
Liver disease, 72, 90, 92, 93, 152, 172, 181, 201, 224; diet and, 118; monitoring, 132
Lumps: checking, 23; removing, 104; vaccine, 194
Lyme disease, 49, 50, 174; vaccination for, 83, 191, 192

McConnell, Patricia, 183
Medication information sheets (MIS), 130, 137
Medications, v, xxix, xxxvii, 19, 20, 21, 32, 71, 205; antianxiety, 182; behavior-modifying, 10; counterfeit, 134; ear, 134, 135; emergency, 206; estrogen-based, 132; eye, 134, 135; flea, 82, 83, 84, 85, 101; giving, xxxvii, 129, 130, 133, 134–135, 159; incontinence, 132; labels for, 132, 133, 134; multiple, 133–134; pain, xxxvii, 102, 104, 131, 158, 159, 160, 162, 177; preventive, 59, 60; side effects of, 129, 132, 164; wrong, 129–130
Methicillin-resistant *Staphylococcus intermedius* (MRSA), 223
Microalbuminuria, 214
Microchipping, 83, 85, 104, 160, 177
Misinformation, xii, xxvii, xxx, 9, 20, 143, 171, 182, 194; money matters and, 99
Molecular therapy, 21
Money issues, 39, 99–108
Monitoring, 27, 46, 132, 213, 214
Monkey pox, 224

National Association of Boards of Pharmacy, 134
National Training Laboratory Institute for Applied Behavior Science, xxiv
Neoplasia, 15
Nestlé Purina PetCare, 116, 117
Neurological development, lack of, 81
Neurological disease, 222
Neurotransmitters, mood elevation and, xviii
Neutering, 80, 84–85, 158–159, 163, 198, 206, 212; benefits of, 160; cancer and, 23
North American Veterinary Nutraceutical Council, 118
Nutraceuticals, 113–120, 140
Nutrients, 118, 217
Nutrition, 21, 29, 79, 80, 83, 113–120, 141, 192, 211, 212, 213; counseling for, 204; dental, 26; obesity and, 198
Obedience training, xxv, 80, 83, 135

Obesity, vii, 150, 151, 158, 200, 201; arthritis and, 217; diet and, 116; life expectancy and, 197; risk of, 114, 198
Oral cavity, disorders of, 217
Oral ulcers, 217
Orthopedic problems, vii, 73
Osteoarthritis (OA), 71, 73

Pain, xii, 28, 71, 72, 79, 120, 151, 158–159; joint, 73; managing, 17, 25, 158, 160, 164; post-surgical, 167
Pancreatitis, 213
Parasites, 43–51, 59, 66, 67, 84; blood, 43; external, 224; fun facts about, 68; intestinal, 44, 65–69, 83, 190; preventing, 60, 61, 66, 205; treating, 68, 149; vaccinations and, 149
Parvovirus, 89, 190
Patience, 20, 144, 179, 184; importance of, xxxi–xxxii
Payments, 35, 104–105, 215; agreement form for, 112; arranging, 104, 106, 107; methods of, xiii, 99, 100–101, 106, 107; understanding, 108
Periodontal disease, xxi, 25, 26, 27, 29, 30, 31, 213, 217
Permethrin, 45
Pet foods, xii; calories from, 114–115, 200; changing, 115–116; diet, 199; OTC, 119–120; post-surgical, 169; premium, 113; quality control for, 114, 119; recommending, 116, 141
Pharmacy, 129–135, 205
Phenylpropanolamine, 132, 182
Phone shoppers, xxxii, 172, 173, 175
Pill poppers, 129, 135
Plaque buildup, 26, 172
Poison control hotlines, 40
Polymerase chain reaction (PCR) tests, 90
Polyuria polydipsia (PU/PD), 181
Prescriptions, xxxvi, 45, 130
Probiotics, 113, 114, 115, 118
Procedures, xxix, 102, 106, 157; explaining, 38, 105; high-tech, 203–208; items necessary for, 110; refusing, 143; understanding, 31
Products, selling, xxviii–xxix, 124, 126, 127
Professionalism, importance of, xv–xvi, 38, 77, 78, 105
Prostaglandins, 120
Proteinuria, 214
Protocols, xxviii, 49, 93, 193, 214; developing, xii–xiii, 215; emergency, 40; kitten, 84–85; parasite, 66; puppy, 82–83; vaccination, 79, 189, 191, 194
Protozoa, 67
Puppies, caring for, 77–85
Pyoderma, 83
Pyometra, 160
Pyrethrin, 45

Quality of life, 17, 21, 30, 197, 202
Questions, xxxv, 78, 151, 181, 182, 211; answering, 125, 140–141, 159, 173–177, 216, 225; asking, xx, 124, 125, 139–143, 158; behavior, 179, 181; phone shopper, 173–177

Rabies, 79, 221, 225; vaccination for, 83, 85, 191, 192, 193, 222
Radiographs, 27, 71, 103, 164, 182, 203, 206
Rat bite fever, 224
Recommendations, xiii, xx, 103, 143, 193; finances and, 105–106; following, xviii, xxvii; health-care, 211–218; reinforcing, 192
Red blood cell count, 96
Renal failure, 142, 181
Repetition, 8, 28, 100, 200; importance of, xxiii–xxv, 16, 126, 161, 162
Resilin, 44
Resorptive lesions, 29, 31
Respiratory diseases, 63, 190
Responsibility, xiv, 40, 42, 178
Ringworm, 50, 207, 225
Risk management, 149–153, 155, 214
Risks, viii, 17, 139, 212; detailing, 105; de-

termining, 153; prioritizing, 150, 151; reducing, 149, 182
Rocky Mountain spotted fever, 49
Roundworms, 60, 65, 66, 68, 221, 222, 225

Sales, xvii, 176, 179; OTC, 123–127, 153
Salmonella, 223, 225
SaME, 118
Sarcoptic mites, 50, 221, 224, 225
Scabies, 225
Scaling, 26, 30
Schwartz, Marti Ann, xv, xvi, xxvi
Screening, vi, xxv, xxxv, 90, 91, 92, 149, 150, 212, 214; cancer, 23; urine, 213; wellness, 101
Seasonal affective disorder, xviii
Seizures, 45, 222
Senior pets, 151; care for, 211–212, 216–217; health-care recommendations for, 211–218
Separation anxiety, 5
Septicemia, 217
Service, xv, 102, 104, 175, 205; deferring/refusing, 143; payment for, 107; protocols, xii–xiii; selling, xvii, xxviii–xxix, 127
Shampoo, 123, 125, 127, 216–217
Shirmer tear test (STT), 214
Skills, vi, viii, xi, xxxi
Skin problems, 50, 66, 120, 205, 225
Socialization, 7, 8, 9–10, 78, 81, 135, 175, 190
Spay/Neuter Your Pet (SNYP), 161
Spaying, 23, 80, 84, 158–159, 160, 163, 198, 206, 212, 214
Splenectomy, 21, 102
Spraying, 8, 9, 161, 181
Stomatitis, 217
Stool checks, xii, 66, 85, 104
Stool samples, 65, 67, 175, 205
Streptococcus bacteria, 223, 224
Stress, xviii, 10, 19, 79, 232
Submissive wetting, 80, 181

Surgery, 103, 124, 131, 157, 203, 204, 206; care following, 169; communications about, 162, 163; cost of, 175, 177; decision making about, 167; estimates for, 105, 110–111; noninvasive, 159; packs, 176; release forms, 163; risks of, 160; things to consider for, 163, 164, 166–167; vaccinations and, 175, 176

Tapeworms, 43–44, 65, 68
Tartar, 26, 32, 116, 141
Teaching, v, vi, xxii, xxix–xxx, 7, 10, 48, 49, 80, 150
Technology, 45, 62, 89, 90, 203–208
Teeth, 32, 81; cleaning, 26; extracting, 31, 203
Telephone skills, xiii, 171–179
Tests, vi, 90, 143, 157, 206; breed-specific, 90, 160, 162; fecal, 58, 68, 101, 177, 214, 223; screening, 212; senior, 90, 91, 97–98; temperament, 212; thyroid, 150; urine, 117; wellness, 92, 98, 214
Thermoregulation, 217
Thrombocytopenia, 49
Thyroid, 9, 90; abnormalities, 89, 201
Ticks, 43–51, 204, 224
Titers, 193, 194
Tooth resorption, 25
Toothbrushing, xxiv, 28, 29, 83, 141
Toothpastes, xxiv, 29, 82, 84
Tours, hospital, 203, 205, 206
Toxoplasmosis, 222, 223, 225
Training, xiii, 5–10, 80, 182; problems with, vii, 5, 6
Treatment, v, xxxiii, 4, 45, 173, 205, 213; appreciation for, xxvii; decision making about, 17–21; descriptions of, xxxvii; estimates for, 110–111; plans, xxxiii, xxxv, 19, 139, 182; withholding, 29–30
Treats, 29, 115, 117, 198, 200
Triponin, 214
Tumors, 9, 160, 161, 206, 217

Ultrasounds, viii, xxi, 182, 203–208, 214
Understanding, xxxiv, xxxv, xxxvii, 103, 173
Upper respiratory signs, 139, 145
Urinalysis, 150, 152, 214
Urinary disorders, 102, 114, 181–185, 198, 205
Urination, 181; problems with, 182, 183, 184–185
U.S. Food and Drug Administration (FDA), 118, 134

Vaccinations, v, viii, xii, xiii, xxix, xxxv, xxxviii, 2, 78, 83, 84, 85, 104, 151, 177, 189–196, 204, 211, 222; booster, 189, 193, 194; calls about, 173, 175; cancer, 21; importance of, 149; information on, 24; overdue, 178; protocols for, 79, 189, 191, 194; selling, 174; surgery and, 175, 176; tick-borne diseases and, 50
Vaginitis, 83, 181
Value statements, 124–125, 126, 153, 172, 173, 215
Veterinary Oral Health Council (VOHC), 28, 29
Veterinary Pet Insurance (VPI), 181
Veterinary teams, xxx, 231; care by, xxxi, 37; communication by, v, 157; education of, xxviii; interactions by, 215, 216; supporting/consoling, 144
Veterinary technicians, vi, xxv, xxix, 141, 142
Videos, xxviii, 6, 39, 92, 201

Viral diseases, 193
Visual learners, xxii
Vitamins, 140, 141, 199
Vomiting, 17, 45, 62, 63, 66, 67, 68, 102, 116, 139, 194
Von Willebrand's disease, 163

Weight, cancer and, 23
Weight control, vii, 197–202, 212, 213
Weight loss, 116, 197, 200, 201, 202
Wellness programs, xvii, 79, 95, 124, 215
West Nile virus, 221
Whipworm eggs, 68
White blood count (WBC), 90, 96
White, Linda M., 9
Wilson, James F., 32
Wisconsin Cat Club, 183
Wisconsin Veterinary Medical Association, xxvi

X-rays, viii, 30, 32, 102, 163, 173, 177, 203–208, 213, 214
Xylitol, 115

"Yes" options, xxxi, 91

Ziglar, Zig, viii
Zoonotic diseases, viii, 221–226, 228–229, 231

ABOUT THE AUTHOR

Nan Boss, DVM, grew up in the Chicago suburbs and earned both her bachelor's degree in biology and her veterinary degree at the University of Illinois. She practiced at a mixed practice for two and a half years before moving to the Milwaukee area. After a year doing equine medicine, she settled into small animal practice, and currently owns the Best Friends Veterinary Center in Grafton, Wisconsin.

Frustrated by the lack of good client education tools, Dr. Boss developed a complete set of handout materials to use in her practice, including sets on the care of puppies, kittens, adult dogs and cats, and geriatric dogs and cats. Her handouts also cover topics such as dry skin in pets, flea treatments, traveling with pets, pet allergies, and many other common pet owner concerns. Her complete set of handouts, compiled in *The Client Education Notebook: Customized Client Education Materials to Use in Your Own Practice*, is available from AVLS-PetCom. Her team training materials, *How We Do Things Here*, were published by AAHA Press in 2008, and she has published articles in numerous veterinary publications.

In her spare time, Dr. Boss is active in several veterinary organizations and speaks for veterinary groups on client-education topics, team training and development, conflict resolution, medical record keeping, and wellness program development. She shares a 120-year-old house with Bob, her husband of 25 years, as well as three rescued cats and a rescued dog.